PERSONAL PERSISTENCE, IDENTITY DEVELOPMENT, AND SUICIDE: A STUDY OF NATIVE AND NON-NATIVE NORTH AMERICAN ADOLESCENTS

Michael J. Chandler
Christopher E. Lalonde
Bryan W. Sokol
Darcy Hallett

WITH COMMENTARY BY
James E. Marcia

Willis F. Overton
Series Editor

MONOGRAPHS OF THE SOCIETY FOR RESEARCH IN CHILD DEVELOPMENT
Serial No. 273, Vol. 68, No. 2, 2003

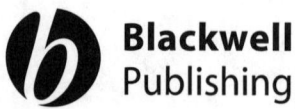 Boston, Massachusetts   Oxford, United Kingdom

EDITOR
WILLIS F. OVERTON
Temple University

EDITORIAL ASSISTANT
MARGARET BERRY
Temple University

CONSULTING EDITORS FOR THE MONOGRAPHS (2003)

Eric Amsel
Weber State University

William Arsenio
Wesleyan University

Stephanie M. Carlson
University of Washington

W. Andrew Collins
University of Minnesota

Jeremy Carpendale
Simon Frasier University

Michael Cole
University of California at San Diego

Doris Entwisle
John Hopkins University

Kurt Fischer
Harvard University

Nancy Galambos
University of Alberta

Elizabeth Gershoff
Columbia University

Uwe Gielen
St. Francis College

William Graziano
Purdue University

Joan Grusec
University of Totongo

John Grych
Marquette University

D. Zachary Hambrick
Michigan State University

Penny Hauser-Cram
Boston College

Charles Helwig
University of Toronto

Grayson N. Holmbeck
Layola University Chicago

Jenny Jenkins
University of Toronto

Charles Kalish
University of Wisconsin

Paul Klaczynski
Pennsylvania State University

Robert E. Larzeler
University of Nebraska

Sherri Levy
State University of New York at Stony Brook

Catherine Lord
University of Michigan

James Marcia
Simon Fraser University

Gayla Margolin
University of Southern California

Ann McGillicuddy-De Lisi
Lafayette College

Lou Moses
University of Oregon

Ulrich Mueller
Pennsylvania State University

Yuko Munakata
University of Colorado

Larry Nucci
University of Illinois at Chicago

Kimberly Powlishta
Washington University (St. Louis, MO)

Mary Jo Ratterman
Franklin & Marshall College

Richard W. Robins
University of California

Sally Rogers
University of California (The Mind Institute)

Diane Ruble
New York University

James Russell
Cambridge University

Judi Smetana
University of Rochester

Bryan Sokol
University of British Columbia

Janet Spence
Professor Emeritus University of Texas

Zolinda Stoneman
University of Georgia

Sue Taylor Parker
Sonoma State University

Ross Thompson
University of Nebraska

PERSONAL PERSISTENCE, IDENTITY DEVELOPMENT, AND SUICIDE: A STUDY OF NATIVE AND NON-NATIVE NORTH AMERICAN ADOLESCENTS

CONTENTS

ABSTRACT	vii
I. INTRODUCTION	1
II. THE ANTINOMY OF SAMENESS AND CHANGE	5
III. ON SELF-CONTINUITY AND ITS DEVELOPMENTAL VICISSITUDES—WHAT YOUNG PEOPLE HAVE TO SAY ABOUT THE PARADOX OF SAMENESS AND CHANGE	19
IV. SELF-CONTINUITY AND YOUTH SUICIDE	50
V. FROM SELF-CONTINUITY TO CULTURAL CONTINUITY—ABORIGINAL YOUTH SUICIDE	61
VI. CULTURE AS A SET POINT IN THE CHOICE BETWEEN NARRATIVIST AND ESSENTIALIST SELF-CONTINUITY WARRANTING PRACTICES	77
VII. CONCLUSIONS	108
APPENDIX SAMPLE QUESTIONS FROM THE PERSONAL PERSISTENCE INTERVIEW	118
REFERENCES	120
ACKNOWLEDGMENTS	129

COMMENTARY

TREADING FEARLESSLY: A COMMENTARY ON PERSONAL PERSISTENCE, IDENTITY DEVELOPMENT, AND SUICIDE *James E. Marcia*	131
CONTRIBUTORS	139
STATEMENT OF EDITORIAL POLICY	140

ABSTRACT

CHANDLER, MICHAEL J.; LALONDE, CHRISTOPHER E.; SOKOL, BRYAN W.; and HALLETT, DARCY. Personal Persistence, Identity Development, and Suicide: A Study of Native and Non-Native North American Adolescents. *Monographs of the Society for Research in Child Development*, 2003, **68** (2, Series No. 273)

The cross-cultural program of research presented here is about matters of temporal persistence—*personal* persistence and *cultural* persistence—and about solution strategies for solving the paradox of "sameness-in-change." The crux of this paradox resides in the fact that, on threat of otherwise ceasing to be recognizable as a self, all of us must satisfy at least two constitutive conditions. The first of these is that selves are obliged to keep moving or die, and, so, must continually change. The second is that selves must also somehow remain the same, lest all notions of moral responsibility and any commitment to an as yet unrealized future become nonsensical. Although long understood as a problem demanding the attention of philosophers, we argue that this same paradox arises in the ordinary course of identity development and dictates the different developmental routes taken by culturally mainstream and Aboriginal youth in coming to the identity-preserving conclusion that they and others are somehow continuous through time.

Findings from a set of five studies are presented. The first and second studies document the development and refinement of a method for parsing and coding what young people say on the topic of personal persistence or self-continuity. Both studies demonstrate that it is not only possible to seriously engage children as young as age 9 or 10 years in detailed and codable discussions about personal persistence, but that their reasoning concerning such matters typically proceeds in an orderly and increasingly sophisticated manner over the course of their early identity development. Our third study underscores the high personal costs of failing to sustain a workable sense of personal persistence by showing that failures to warrant self-continuity are strongly associated with increased suicide risk in adolescence. Study four documents this same relation between continuity and suicide, this time at the macrolevel of whole cultures, and shows that efforts by Aboriginal groups to preserve and promote their culture are associated with dramatic reductions in rates of youth suicide. In the final study we show that different default strategies for resolving the paradox of personal persistence and change—*Narrative* and *Essentialist strategies*—distinctly characterize Aboriginal and non-Aboriginal youth.

I. INTRODUCTION

This *Monograph* is about identity development and the paradox of personal and cultural persistence in the face of inevitable change. It is also about First Nations people (or what some, assuming innocence, still call "Indians") and what causes the young among them to so often take their own lives. But more than anything, it is about continuities—continuities of the self, of others, and even of whole communities—and how it is that young people, both Aboriginal and not, regularly work to understand themselves as surviving time in ways that guarantee a past and a future they can live with and count as their own. (In keeping with common practice in Canada, the term "aboriginal" is used here to refer to indigenous persons in general, whereas "Aboriginal" refers to several specific groups within Canada: Inuit, First Nations, and Métis). All of these enigmatic matters (about personal persistence and youth suicide and cultural continuities) are large-scale, too large to easily fit in this, or even in several monographs. Faced with this limitation, we mean to hold ourselves to an account of just three questions, only two of which are about killing oneself.

The first of these questions turns on the classic paradox of sameness and change. We are doubtlessly all works in progress, obliged to change by the temporally vectored nature of our public and private existence. Still, and just as certainly, if we are to qualify as recognizable instances of what selves are ordinarily taken to be (Cassirer, 1923), we must find ways to interpretively override at least some of these changes by working to make each of the distinctive time slices that together form the archipelago of our life count as belonging timelessly to one and the same person.

Understanding ourselves and others as continuous is not some elective feature of selves that can be taken up or left alone, but needs to be seen instead as a fundamental condition of their actually coming into being. The problem, then, is one of reconciling necessary sameness in the face of constant change. Everyone must negotiate solutions to this problem, often again and again. The open question is: How do we all do it? The answer, as our research aims to show, is: In more and sundry ways than you likely ever imagined possible. Even if we only manage to be clear about this—our major challenge—by successfully lining out how young people (of different ages and different cultures) successfully negotiate and renegotiate the problem of their own "numerical identity," that would be something. As it is, however, stopping here is not an option. It is simply not possible to take the proper measure of young people's various successes in solving the problem of sameness within change without also considering the likely nature and costs of their possible failures.

Problems two and three are both about these costs (the personal and the collective price) of failing to get question number one right, and about death incarnate. In particular, question two turns on the well-known fact that adolescents and young adults are especially at risk of dropping the thread of their own continuous existence. One particularly heartbreaking correlate of such failures is, as we will argue, the alarming frequency with which teenagers and young adults both attempt to take and succeed at taking their own lives in numbers that are out of all proportion to the size of their age population—by various counts, at rates anywhere from 3 to 300 times those characteristic of other age groups (Meehan, Lamb, & Saltzman, 1992). The numbers we can compute. What we cannot understand is how they could actually bring themselves to do it. How could they throw away their lives and all of our futures, often over seeming trifles that (should they somehow succeed in surviving to tell the tale) will later be judged to scarcely matter? Suicides, especially youth suicides, almost never seem to make sense. The research to be reported here was predicated on the assumption that coming to a better understanding of the changing ways in which young people struggle, and sometimes fail, to understand themselves as personally persistent may provide a key to the problem of youth suicide.

What ties the notion of personal persistence to the problem of youth suicide, as we mean to demonstrate, is that, without some means of counting oneself as continuous in time, there simply would be no reason to show appropriate care and concern for one's own future well-being. When we, as adults, contemplate our own demise, the dead person that we ordinarily imagine on the floor is decisively us. Young people, it too often happens, are not like that. Rather, handicapped by an ephemeral sense of their own personal persistence, they often lose the thread that tethers together their past, present, and future, leaving them open to the risk of suicide. This, in short, is the thrust of some of the research to be reported here, research that explores the relation between individual and collective efforts to achieve a workable sense of self-continuity or durable identity on the one hand, and suicidal behaviors in both culturally mainstream and Aboriginal youth on the other.

Our *third* and final question is much like the second, and differs mainly in that it concerns the special problem of suicide among the world's

Aboriginal youth. In Canada, where our research was conducted, First Nations and other Aboriginal youth reportedly take their own lives at rates that are said to be higher than that of any culturally identifiable group in the world (Kirmayer, 1994), and these rates are closely matched by their aboriginal counterparts throughout the Americas (Resnik & Dizmang, 1971) and beyond (Carsten, 2000). How does it happen that death is the preferred alternative for so many Aboriginal youth? Again, our plan will be to make the case that problems in negotiating a sense of continuity (not just personal but also collective or cultural continuity) lie at the heart of this third question. As our research will show, whole Aboriginal communities that have succeeded, against mounting odds, in rehabilitating their badly savaged cultures, not only apparently salvage their past and harness their future but, along the way, also manage to successfully insulate their youth from the risk of suicide.

Despite the fact that this *Monograph* is meant to address the problem of youth suicide, both at the individual and community levels, this is neither the right rhetorical place to begin nor the place where this program of research actually began. Rather, suicide, like so much of what befalls young persons, can only make interpretive sense if we first situate such self-destructive acts in their proper developmental context. That is, what needs to be understood first is how most young people ordinarily succeed in surviving the ravages of time with their lives and their identities still intact. If we understood this, if we could get a better conceptual grip on the procedural means by which developing persons ordinarily manage to own their past and commit to their future, then there would be grounds for some hope of making real sense out of those exceptions to the more general rule who undertake to kill themselves.

This, at least, is how our research began more than a decade ago. Then, as now, we wanted to know how young persons gradually succeed in coming to a defensible understanding of their own temporal coherence—an understanding that both allows them to own their past and permits them a proper measure of care and concern about the future well-being of the self they are en route to becoming.

We will proceed by working our way through a series of five talking points that are each taken up as separate chapters in the pages that follow. As a sort of preview to these main themes of our research, here, in brief, are the matters that we mean to speak to in turn.

First, as a way of beginning, we will say something synoptic about what is usually intended by talk about self-continuity or personal persistence, and we will try and make clear why failing to understand oneself as a singularity—as a diachronically continuous or "numerically identical" self that deserves to be counted only once—risks costing each of us a sense of responsibility for our own past and a sense of commitment to our own future.

Second, we will (a) describe the methods and procedures we developed during our effort to measure young people's assumptions about their own and others' continuity or personal persistence and (b) present a series of developmental findings that spell out how rank-and-file young persons ordinarily grow in sophistication as they repeatedly try to solve the problem of their own personal continuity in time.

Third, we will discuss why failing to negotiate some serviceable way of grasping one's own personal persistence works to impair that ordinary sense of care and concern that helps to ensure our future well-being. We illustrate these prospects by turning attention to the problem of youth suicide, and by demonstrating how unresolved problems in the ordinary process of warranting a sense of personal sameness can help in accounting for the otherwise poorly understood epidemic of suicidal behaviors known to occur during adolescence.

Fourth, because there are good reasons to presume that concerns over matters of persistence exist at both individual and group levels of analyses, we undertook a still-building epidemiological study that examines, not *personal* continuity, but *cultural* continuity in British Columbia's Aboriginal Communities. We report a portion of these data that relates the variable success that different Aboriginal communities have had in trying to preserve or promote their own cultures, and the frequency of youth suicide in their communities.

Fifth, and finally, we turn our attention to the comparative study of the course of identity development in Aboriginal, as well as non-Aboriginal youth, and provide details of our ongoing efforts to characterize the distinctive self-continuity warranting practices, not only of young persons from Canada's "cultural mainstream," but also from two First Nations communities.

II. THE ANTINOMY OF SAMENESS AND CHANGE

In naming, as we did in our introductory remarks, the so-called paradox of sameness within change as the first of several questions to be addressed, the bare beginnings of a case was made for insisting, as we now mean to insist all the more, that *persistence* is foundational to, or constitutive of, what it ordinarily means to be a self or person. Although we intend for this claim to have the automatic feel of intuitive rightness, so much of what follows presupposes its legitimacy that a more serious attempt at persuasion needs to be made in order to bring you along with us in this conviction. We mean to do this (a) by assuaging any lingering doubts you might have about the inevitability of personal change; (b) by convincing you, if you need more convincing, that any account of selves that did not make adequate provision for understanding each of us as somehow possessing real sameness (or at least persistence) through time would end up striking us as fundamentally nonsensical (Luckman, 1979); and (c) by calling into serious question the deeply suspect postmodern fable that characterizes all commitments to the continuity of selfhood as an unfortunate byproduct of supposedly discredited Enlightenment thought.

Of all of these tasks, the success of the one meant to further convince you that change is near the top of any list of life's necessary constants seems least in doubt. Because selfhood is everywhere acknowledged to be temporally vectored (Gallagher, 1998), no one seriously doubts that change is real. Our bodies change, our beliefs and desires along with our projects and our commitments and our relationships all change, often seemingly beyond all recognition. All ironies aside, change needs to be counted as a permanent fixture of our existence, and so seen to lie at the heart of subjectivity (Gallagher). If it did not, then, as Unger (1975) reminded us, "we could make sense of neither the experience of innovation in the lives of individuals, nor novelty in the flow of human history" (p. 56).

This talk of change is, of course, only half of a matched pair. Here is the other shoe. Except for the occasional scorched-earth postmodernist (Chandler, 1997), no one boldly believes that everything is change and polysemic flux (Chandler, 2001). This follows because change, though no doubt inevitable, is rarely exceptionless. If this were not so, if nothing about us remained the same to ensure our reliable reidentification, then life as we ordinarily understand it would simply have no followable meaning.

With both halves of the antinomy firmly in place, the classic paradox of sameness and change is set—a paradox whose hoped for resolution is, as we will argue, foundational to any workable conception of self- or personhood.

PARADOX AND RESOLUTION

Although it remains possible to playfully imagine that either sameness or change is a mere illusion, or that each is the negative correlative contrary of the other, it is not possible to seriously manage one's life on such either/or assumptions. Instead, driven by the absurdity of the consequence to which such "split positions" (Overton, 1998) inevitably lead, our common contemporary obligation is broadly taken to be that of working out how selves "can embody both change and permanence simultaneously" (Fraisse, 1963, p. 10). That is, if neither personal sameness nor personal change can be made to work alone, then we clearly need to arrive at some viable way of understanding selves as both simultaneously fixed and ongoing. This is so because, as Strawson (1999) put it, there is "a deep presumption that if one is arguing for the existence of the mental self, one is arguing for something that exists for a substantial period of time ... a diachronic singleness [that] allows one to regard the series of thoughts and experiences that make up one's life as the thoughts [and experiences] of a single self" (p. 10). In short, although our lives are composed of innumerable episodes, each with its own viewpoint and focus and role, we are, nevertheless, all seemingly geared in whatever ways are necessary to allow us "to hold various things constant" (Turner, 1996, p. 124), and to "see ourselves as transcending our singularities" (p. 134) in whatever fashion is required to render such different time-slices as all episodes in the career of one and the same person.

This idea that self-continuity is an ineradicable feature of personhood and identity is among the oldest of our old ideas. For example, in the first chapter of Book Two of his *Physics*, Aristotle stated that "animals differ from what is not naturally constituted in that each of these [living] things has within it a principle of change and of staying unchanged" (cited in Wiggins, 1980, pp. 88–89). More than a millennium and a half later, Locke (1694/1956) similarly wrote in *An Essay Concerning Human Understanding* that, in order to meet even the minimal condition for selfhood, it is necessary to consider one's self "as the same thinking thing in different times and places." Nearer to our own time, William James (1910) also made continuity a cornerstone of his conception of selfhood, as have a long list of more contemporary philosophers such as Cassirer (1923), who spoke of "temporal unity," Chisholm (1971), who talked of "intact persistence," and Strawson (1999), who emphasized what he called our "diachronic singleness." These accounts and those of many other contemporary philosophers (e.g., see Harré, 1979; Hirsch, 1976; MacIntyre, 1977; Parfit, 1971; Rorty, 1976; Taylor, 1991; Wiggins, 1980), along with a similar complement of touchstone psychological theorists (e.g., Erikson, 1968; Perry, 1976; Piaget, 1968), share the common conclusion that being seen to remain self-same across the various phases of our temporal existence needs to be counted as a constitutive condition for being recognized as any sort of person at all (Chandler, Lalonde, & Sokol, 2000; Lewis & Ferrari, 2001). All of this, and more, adds up to a long brief in support of what Flanagan (1996, p. 65) has called our self-imposed "one self to a customer rule."

PASTS AND POSSIBILITIES

> *The past and the possible [are] the modalities for self-making.*
> E. Ochs & L. Capps, "Narrative Authenticity," 1997

The claim that the earlier and later manifestations of a life must somehow count as belonging timelessly to one and the same continuant (van Inwagen, 1990) needs to be seen as true, not simply because so many important people say that it is so, but for at least two persuasive reasons, one of which is quintessentially historical and *backward referring*, the other *forward anticipating* and so all about our own as yet unrealized futures. As William James put it, a life is like a "saddleback" or a "skiff" moving through time with a bow as well as a stern (cited in Flanagan, 1996).

First, and with reference to things off the stern, each of us needs to be understood as temporally persistent because, if we could not count (or reidentify) ourselves and others as the same continuous and "numerically identical" individuals across time—that is, if we could not successfully link up earlier time-slices of our lives with the persons we have since become—then social life as we ordinarily understand it would come to a standstill. This follows for the reason that, in its backward-referring aspect, self-continuity is no less than a moral, political, legal, and economic imperative (Whittaker, 1992). Without a way of owning our own past, our concepts of moral responsibility would be emptied of meaning (Rorty, 1973), all grounds for owning up to legal obligations or liabilities would be lost (Whittaker), contracts and debts and promises would all fly out the same window, all prospects for a just and moral world would evaporate, and Judgment Day would simply go out of business. How could there be a heaven or hell, where those with a history of good and evil are meant to languish, if it were not possible to understand ways in which each of us legitimately owns his or her own past (Flanagan, 1996)?

Much the same proves to be true of our own as yet unrealized *futures*. Selves, in MacIntyre's words (1984), are on a perpetual "quest." That is, as Bakhtin (1986, p. 26) argued, we are built up not only out of "remnants of the past but also from rudiments and tendencies of the future," rudiments that give "a sense to one's life as having a direction towards what one not yet is" (Taylor, 1988, p. 48). Seen, then, from the bow, we behave as we do in the anxious anticipation that, in Unger's (1975) words, we will later become the natural inheritors of our own "just deserts." In support of the same point, Flanagan (1996) argued that "As beings in time, we are navigators. We care how our lives go" (p. 67). Why, if all this were not so, would anyone stop smoking or go on a diet or bother to get an education? We forgo short-run pleasures for long-term gain because, among other things, we find it reasonable to suppose that, when all is said and done, the knowledgeable, thin person with healthy lungs would somehow still be us. Similarly (and here we anticipate), why don't we just put ourselves out of our misery whenever the going gets tough? Why should we care one way or another about the well being of the radically changed self we each are en route to becoming? Though we mean to shortly have more to say about these matters, for the moment our point is to remind you that there is a "rub," and that "what doth make cowards of us all" is, more often than not, the certain conviction that the person who would automatically bear the consequence of all such attempts at suicide or self-injury would again be us.

For all of the backward-referring and forward-anticipating reasons just offered, then, the Janus-faced notion of personal persistence is ordinarily (many would say "universally") understood to be an immanent providence at work in the whole of human affairs (Shotter, 1984).

AGAINST PERSISTENCE

There are those who take umbrage at all claims to the effect that *any* aspect of human nature whatsoever could possibly qualify as somehow transsituational or transhistorical or otherwise be part of a broader "human nature" (for a review, see Chandler, 1999). The general line of argumentation thrown up by such postmodern critics (e.g., Lampinen & Odegard, 2000) involves pointing to real or imagined hard cases in which the putative "singularity of life" (Turner, 1996, p. 116) is supposedly brought into deep question. What, it is proposed, if you fell into a copy machine, or your body stayed in place while your brain was teleported to Houston Central? What if you became amnesic, or suffered from a multiple personality disorder? More realistically, what if you underwent some identity crisis, or simply thought and behaved differently at home and at the office? Though none of these matters are without interest or philosophical import, they do all somehow miss the point. As Rorty (1973) pointed out, "talk of psychological fusion, or multiple role identification, or demonic [dis]possession [all] presuppose a person to whom all of these are referred, parts of whose continuous story they are, or to whom they all belong" (p. 74). That is, whatever divisive things may be going on in the real or imagined minds of those who are said to suffer such assaults to their singularity, the work of having singled them out for special attention presupposes having already identified the persistent person whose changeable experience is at issue—persons or selves who we (and often they) invariably regard as being under some sort of misapprehension or delusion. Here, as elsewhere, then, the point of such postmodern criticisms continues to be blunted as a consequence of repeatedly bumping into one such performative contradiction after another (Chandler, 1999).

ALTERNATIVE APPROACHES TO CONTINUITY

Resting as it does on more than 2000 years of Euro-American intellectual history, and backed, as it consequently is, by our contemporary version of common sense, the ordinary conviction that selves are necessarily continuous strikes most as true enough. Still, more is likely required if you are to go away persuaded, as we intend, that perenniality is actually an exceptionless design feature of any and all workable conceptions of selfhood. In short order (and more particularly in chap. III) we will report on a large-scale empirical attempt to illustrate how it is that, almost without exception, young people of different ages and distinctive sociocultural backgrounds are actually prepared to spend an inordinate amount of energy attempting to, and generally succeeding at, answering such continuity questions for themselves. Before coming to this evidence, however, it seems prudent to first try to anticipate at least some of the self-continuity warranting strategies that the young participants in our research might take.

A LITERATURE IN ABSENTIA

Despite the fact that a long list of touchstone philosophers and theologians dating back to the very beginnings of Western intellectual history have promoted the importance of continuity as a constitutive condition of self- and personhood, and not withstanding the fact that key figures in psychology's more recent history such as James and Erikson have made convictions about one's personal persistence a central pillar of their theorizing about identity development, actual empirical studies meant to detail the course by means of which young people arrive at increasingly mature beliefs about their own temporal persistence are unaccountably few. There are a few studies in which young (mostly preschool) children are queried about the persistence of artifacts and living things, sometimes including themselves (e.g., Gutheil & Rosengren, 1996; Hall, 1998; Hart, Maloney & Damon, 1987; Peevers, 1987). These relatively isolated studies are, however, largely given over to contrasting "individual" and "kind" persistence, and have generally failed to initiate programmatic efforts to explore the course and consequences of early ideas about self-continuity.

There is also a small but influential clinical literature that documents some of what can go wrong in the lives of those who evidently lose themselves in time, or who suffer some catastrophic failure in their attempts to vouchsafe their own diachronic singularity (Strawson, 1999). Associated writings by Erikson (1968), Marcia (1966), and other like-minded self theorists (e.g., Fromm, 1970) regularly acknowledge, but rarely elaborate on, the importance of personal persistence in explaining the identity crises of adolescents and other transitional groups. Spotty thoughts about sameness in time also similarly concern those who study various sorts of displaced persons, as they do for those interested in amnesia and persons with so-called multiple personality disorders (Hacking, 1995, 1999). Though all of this is certainly important, it is *not* the same thing as a direct frontal attack on the larger problem of understanding and learning how to measure the particular ways in which ordinary people, especially young, ordinary people, generally succeed but sometimes fail in hammering out appropriate criteria for personal persistence, or sameness within change.

The closest thing available to addressing such a developmental question exists in the literature concerned with what has come to be called *psychological essentialism* (Medin, 1989), a literature that from a certain remote viewing distance might be seen to be reasonably on target. DeVries (1969), for example, outfitted available cats with a dog or rabbit mask, and then put questions to young preschoolers about the persistence of feline identity. Similarly, Aboud and Ruble (1987) persuaded groups of young Jewish preschool children to speculate about the continuity of their religious/ethnic identity after first obliging them to put on "Eskimo" [sic] costumes. In much the same vein, but for rather different reasons, Keil (1989), Gelman (1999), and Medin (1989), among others (e.g., Wellman,

1990) documented the emergence of so-called psychological essentialism by pressing young respondents about whether, for example, a skunk would still go on being a skunk after its white stripe was painted out, or, more sinister still, after its "insides were surgically removed." All of this is about persistence after a fashion, but the sort of identity being inquired into in all of these studies was always "kind" identity rather than "individual" identity. That is, when DeVries outfitted cats with masks or Keil spoke of disemboweling skunks the operative question put to the respondents was whether what remained was still a cat or a skunk (i.e., whether these exemplars did or did not persist as members of the same class) and not whether "Tabby" was still "our one and only beloved Tabby" or the skunk was still persistently "Flower," or "Pépé LePu," or whatever particular skunk he or she happened to have been before the surgery. Rather, in such cases, "identity" was taken to be preserved if any transformed object A' was still the same F (where F is a natural kind) as was the original object A before its transformation. However interesting all of this may be, such studies tell us almost nothing about those notions of personal persistence that underlie our social practices of allocating responsibility and dishing out just deserts (Rorty, 1973, p. 269). As Gutheil and Rosengren (1996) pointed out, both human beings and spoons are specific individuals that (within the limits of interest typically operating among those concerned with questions of "kind identity") go right on being tokens of their same "types" through a range of rather trying circumstances. Such studies do all of this, however, without offering much in the way of useful guidance about how one might best proceed in getting at the life-conferring self-continuity warranting practices of children, let alone of adolescents and young adults.

Still closer to our concerns are a few published studies and commentaries meant to explore directly young children's entry level beliefs about personal persistence. Piaget (1968), for example, cited a series of studies undertaken by Voyat that were meant to assess "young children's understanding of the stability of personal identity ... by having them draw pictures of themselves and others at various ages. The claim made on the basis of these efforts is that [before the age of 7] such children already understand that the drawings captured the same individual over time" (Rosengren, Gelman, Kalish, & McCormick, 1991, p. 1304). Others (e.g., Guardo & Bohan, 1971; Gutheil & Rosengren, 1996; Hall, 1998; Inagaki & Sugiyama, 1988) have come to much the same conclusion. What we learn from these several studies is that, by a surprisingly early age, young preschoolers and schoolage children already share with the adults around them the required conviction that at least "things of a natural kind" (as opposed to artifacts) successfully maintain their individual identity across a surprising range of transformations. What we don't learn, and badly need to know, is how such young persons justify or warrant these conclusions, and whether they think about matters of personal persistence differently as a function of their age or circumstance.

Having been generally let down by a research community whose interests are typically elsewhere, and yet still in need of some kind of leg-up in deciding how to best go about measuring young people's changing convictions about personal persistence, we began casting about much more broadly, in the hope of capturing other available best practices and best thoughts about how to proceed in these uncertain matters. What follows is a sampler of some of the more indirect help that we found.

Broadening the Search Pattern

Credible empirical studies concerning beliefs about personal persistence are few, but public pronouncements regarding such matters are not only thick on the contemporary ground but form a deep vein of speculative writings that run to the very core of, at least, Western intellectual history. In fact, a sizeable chunk of the assembled works of Euro-American philosophy can be read as a collection of such beliefs judged worthy of repeating. The open question is how best to make use of such commentaries. Although it would undoubtedly be a mistake to suppose that the ontogeny of our various folk or commonsense beliefs about our diachronic singleness merely recapitulates the historical course of these philosophies, it would also seem equally unlikely that at least some of what has been archivally preserved concerning this topic does not also have its counterpart in some of what lay persons believe and say on the same subject. As such, parts of this recorded history of thoughts about the paradox of sameness within change could potentially serve as a template or "source model" to be used in imagining what ordinary young people might believe about their own numerical identity. On this prospect, effort spent exploring past writings on the theme of personal persistence seemed justified.

Although the range of available "solutions" to the paradox of sameness within change is exceedingly broad, the large bulk of these ideas gravitate toward one or the other pole of what amounts to a standing dichotomy. One of these clusters, characterized here as *Entity* or *Essentialist* positions, involves efforts to marginalize change by attaching special importance to one or more enduring attributes of the self that are imagined to somehow stand outside of or otherwise defeat time. Contrapuntally, the alternative view—solution strategies that we label here as *Relational* or *Narrative*, as opposed to *Essentialist*—proceed in just the opposite direction by throwing their lot in with time and change, and supposing that any residual demands for sameness can be satisfied by pointing to various relational forms that bind together the admittedly distinct time-slices of one's life. On the prospect that something like these classical strategies for navigating the antinomy between sameness and change might find their way into the thoughts of the young people who would participate in our studies, it seems useful to say something more about them in turn.

Essentialism

Essentialist solutions to the problem of personal persistence tend to be favored by those whose metaphysical stance leans toward the analytic rather than the holistic (Norenzayan, Choi, & Nisbett, 1999), the paradigmatic and propositional as opposed to the discursive and historical (Bruner, 1986), the taxonomic in lieu of the schematic (Mandler, 1984), the monistic instead of the dialogical (Hermans, 1996), and the universal or transcendental in contrast to the local or indigenous (Habermas, 1985). Their ambitions tend to favor truth rather than sincerity (Lightfoot, 1997), and their commitment is to the strong claim that all objects, selves included, necessarily possess some timeless core of persistent sameness, some material or transcendental center or atemporal "indelible stain" that stands outside of time (Shalom, 1985) or is otherwise immune to change (Brockelman, 1985).

Of the two views, the Essentialist position is the more venerable, or at least this is regularly said to be true in the context of Western or Euro-American thought. As Schlesinger (1977) put it, "the ancient philosophers" (meaning, ancient Western Philosophers such as Plato) regularly insisted that "being was given once and for all, complete and perfect, in an ultimate system of essences" (p. 271). Clear remnants of such lingering Platonism may have grown rather harder to detect after being filtered through successive generations of Western thought (Smith, 1988), but certain signature constants remain. The kernel idea common to all subspecies of this Essentialist view is that there actually is a kernel idea, some enduring something (DNA, ego, spirit, soul) that, as William James (1891) derisively put it, "stand[s] behind the passing states of consciousness and our always shifting ways of being" (p. 196) and successfully vouchsafes our identities by immobilizing or negating or otherwise defeating time.

As they obviously must, champions of Essentialism recognize that time and all that it contains constantly picks at the threads of whatever sort of identity we have been carefully stitching up. Nevertheless, and ordinarily well before we threaten to come entirely apart at the seams, there still remains, it is argued, some persistent essential kernel of existence that forms the foundation of our identity and from which we can begin the work of knitting back up the raveled sleeve of our persistent selves. As such, Essentialists ordinarily commit their weight to the "sameness" foot, discounting "change" as mere illusion.

Narrativity

Arranged against Essentialism are all of those narrativists, hermeneuticists, and social constructivists, along with an assemblage of presentist historiographers and phenomenologists and champions of all things dialogical, whose generic solution to the problem of personal persistence is to emphasize the connective tissue between things, rather than to imagine the existence of anything enduring or immune to time. As a group (or better yet a collective or community), defenders of this position are ruggedly antimetaphysical and tend to emphasize the extrinsic over the intrinsic (Berzonsky, 1993), process over structure (Ricoeur, 1985), the discursive over the substantial, the relational over the individualistic (Overton, 1998), and the episodic over the semantic (Tulving, 1983). Rejecting out of hand the key foundationalist assumption that the self is naturally rooted in some enduring substance, or illusive transcendental essence, Narrativists generally side with Dennett (1992) in viewing selfhood as something more approximating a "center of narrative gravity." On this more relational account, then, the usual container/substance view of the self typically adopted by Essentialists (Holland, 1997) is discounted in favor of the idea "that the connectedness of life can only be understood through meaning" (Dilthey, 1962, pp. 201–202), meaning conferred on the disparate time-slices of one's life through the fashioning of stories meant to integrate all of one's reconstructed past, present, and anticipated future into some overarching narrative structure (McAdams, Diamond, de St. Aubin, & Mansfield, 1997). In short, in this view, selves are understood to be no more than the narrative embodiment of lives told (Spence, 1982), and they qualify (or fail to qualify) as enduring or persistent to the degree that the stories that are told about them are somehow coherent or followable. This is all imagined possible not only because we are "story-telling animals" (MacIntyre, 1984, p. 201) but because the social and material conditions of human existence themselves are also said to have a fundamentally narrative structure (Kerby, 1991, p. 41).

Narrative, as opposed to Essentialist forms of self-understanding, as we (Chandler, 2000; Chandler & Lalonde, 1998; Chandler et al., 2000) and others (Eakin, 1999) have termed them, are, then, grounded in an entirely different intellectual tradition, a tradition that rejects as mere illusion the supposedly hidden but essential causes imagined by Entity theorists. Instead, the emphasis is on whole-part, or genus-species relations of a sort that renders selves something more like a web or diachronic-patterned relation than an entity, and identities are pictured as more akin to an awareness of process than a test of endurance. As a result, Narrative theorists, or at least those living closest to the radical postmodern edge, tend to promote an altogether more fleeting, aimless, ephemeral, fragmentary sort of "outlaw" notion of selfhood that, by instantly adapting its chameleon ways to whatever contingent circumstances happen to prevail, makes a hero out of change and a goat of sameness.

In their strongest form, such "split" Narrative views (Overton, 1998) amount to a kind of contrary "damn-their-eyes" antiessentialism, in which oppositional forms of Essentialism are simply reduced to Narrativity peevishly stood on its head. Except for the most radical advocates of this position, however, many Narrativists see themselves as being as obliged as the next person to make whatever minimal concessions to sameness are necessary to get recognizable (i.e., reidentifiable) people out the other end. Their typical strategy for accomplishing this, without at the same time reinvoking some tired "idol of the mind" or some "fictive" mental or substantive entity imagined to successfully defy time, is to adopt more phenomenological views in which the stream of ideas that is said to be the mind (Gallagher, 1998) is held out to be "sufficient, in and of itself, to ground the possibility of self-continuity without essence" (Putnam, 1988).

In briefly surveying the available array of such narrativelike or relational accounts, it quickly becomes evident that they are not all of a piece, but instead come in a surprising variety of different flavors. Some, located nearest to the fringe (e.g., Gergen & Gergen, 1983; Harré, 1979) appear at risk of becoming "lost in the tropics of discourse" (Zagorin, 1999, p. 23) by fully equating selves with personal narratives, thereby threatening to completely dissolve personal history into a species of literature. Others (e.g., Car, 1986; Mink, 1969; Ricoeur, 1985; Zagorin, 1999) more cautiously insist that, because our lives are not amenable to just any telling, all of the more radicalized attempts to equate lives and stories only succeed in giving Narrativity a bad name. In either case, however, theorists of all these diverse stripes seem to agree that "it is in telling our stories that we give ourselves an identity" (Ricoeur, 1985, p. 214), and that because nothing of great importance actually does survive time in ways that could effectively warrant our necessary claims for self-continuity anyway, our only possible way to ground personal persistence without "essence" (Putnam, 1988) is to rely on what Flanagan (1996) called "narrative connectedness."

On Choosing Between Narrative and Essentialist Solutions

All that has just been said about Narrative and Essentialist solutions to the problem of personal persistence has emphasized their historical oppositionality. Seen through the eyes of your typical Narratologist, storytelling just *is* the "essential genre" (Flanagan, 1996) or "natural" (MacIntyre, 1984) or "native tongue" (Weintraub, 1975) of the self, or at least represents our "best" and most "privileged" way of giving voice to it (Kerby, 1991). On this exclusionary account, Essentialism is demoted to the status of just another negative byproduct of the Enlightenment, or Romanticism, or high-modernity, and assumed to be present only, if at all, in a handful of Western cultures (Miller, 1996). Essentialists, for their own part, tend to speak with much the same authorial certainty and the same air of presumptive exclusivity, insisting that Essentialism is somehow bred into our bones. Narratologists, they argue, are, at best, practitioners of "mere" rhetoric (Ring, 1987) who have somehow fallen prey to certain recent French fads (Callinicos, 1989).

It is decidedly not our intention to somehow arbitrate these competing metaphysical claims. Our whole point in delving into this maelstrom of divergent opinions is to build up a more "inclusive" (Overton, 1998, p. 112) list of available options or procedural alternatives that individuals and whole communities might draw on and adopt as default strategies in working out for themselves how best to resolve the common paradox of personal sameness within change. What this survey led us to anticipate, and what our interviews with more than 400 adolescents have so far demonstrated, is that some respondents do in fact answer questions about their own personal persistence in ways that are exclusively Essentialist or Narrative in character, and others, in almost equal numbers draw on both of these supposedly oppositional solution strategies as their reading of the situation demands. In either case, what now needs to be made clear is how both the Essentialist and Narrative solution strategies evident in the scholarly literatures surveyed were pressed into service as source models in our own empirical efforts to explore and characterize how individuals and whole cultures actually go about resolving the paradox of sameness and change.

From Theory to Practice

When faced with the task of getting all the way from the disembodied claims that Narrativist and Essentialists theorists tend to make on behalf of the whole of humankind, to whatever concrete, close-to-the-ground details are required to nail down exactly where some particular adolescent boy or girl actually stands on these complex issues, the circumstances of assessment strongly favor Essentialism. That is, if you are convinced that what guarantees your own or others' personal persistence is some more or less concrete something assumed to successfully hide out from time (e.g., if, when asked why you are still one and the same person across the years, you confidently point to your strawberry birthmark), then the job of typecasting your responses is reasonably straightforward. It is possible, of course, that you may be less than clear about what you really do believe, or find yourself at a loss for words. Still, all things being equal, the question is at least clear enough (i.e., "what is it that didn't change?"), as are the usual answers that flood the minds of the typical "lay" Essentialist (e.g., "the lightening bolt scar on my forehead," or "my personality," or "my immortal soul").

By contrast, things are often a good deal less straightforward in the case of those who understand personal persistence in what we have labeled Narrative terms. Possible confusions arise from all quarters. If you interrupt someone who is in the midst of detailing how much they have changed over the years by asking what qualifies them as one and the same person, and if they understand their narration to already be just such an explanation, then they tend to assume that you were simply not paying attention, and cooperation flags. As it is, questions of almost any sort better suit Essentialists, who mean to reveal something hidden. Young Narrativists, by contrast, commonly regard questions meant to quickly get to the bottom of things as interruptions. Such communication difficulties aside, however, the real problem is getting clear about what it could possibly mean to label something as *Narrativelike* and, more than that, getting clear about a Narrative solution strategy of some particular stripe.

Much of the responsibility for the measurement problems just described grows out of the fact that notions about narratives obviously have their origins in intellectual places often remote from mainstream social science (Mishler, 1995)—in literary analysis or semiotics, for example. Consequently, it is easy, as Bell (1990) pointed out, "when importing the term 'narrative' into other disciplines … to confuse its use as an illustrative analogy or metaphor with other more literal definitions, as for example, when talk of narrative order is equated with lived temporality" (p. 172). In short, when we begin to push at the distinction between "narrative" and just about anything else "the whole question of what a narrative might be [often] begins to unravel, often to the extent that so-called narrative discourse might not be distinguishable from any other linguistic act" (McQuillan, 2000, p. 6). What about mere description, or argumentation, or exposition, which, along with narration, are classically said (Riessman, 1993) to box the compass on the full range of discursive modes? What about "Pass the salt?" or "Help!" that are said by some to constitute narratives (McQuillan, 2000)? Surely we are not after all of that. Rather, what interests us here about Narrativity is its reputed ability (along with that of Essentialism) "to make sense out of change and time [by] extracting patterns out of events that have no necessary teleological order of their own"—to impose "a continuous account upon fundamentally discontinuous data" (Freeman, 1984, p. 10). If, as we are quick to agree, something very much like this, something like laying bare the so-called structure of narrative argumentation, is what we are after, then we need not move too far into the troubled and deeply contested, definitional waters that surround the use of these terms (Danziger, 1997, p. 148). Instead, while attempting to avoid some of the hazards posed by what Bell (1990, p. 172) described as the "rich charge of suggestiveness" that surrounds the contemporary use of the term "narrativity," we mean to pursue its relevance to the storied ways in which many young people attempt to link up the various time-slices of their lives, and still leave the door open for other distinctive solution strategies meant to answer questions about personal persistence that don't automatically qualify as being yet another narrative form.

However sharp we make the distinction between Essentialist and Narrative approaches to the problem of self-continuity, it has become a good deal sharper than it was more than a decade ago when this program of research began, and when the participants in our studies, along with their responses, were primarily of Euro-American descent. In the interim we have become alert to the prospect that some of what adolescents had to say about personal persistence is better understood as a good Narrative than a bad Essentialist effort. How we came to this more inclusive view is detailed in chapter III.

III. ON SELF-CONTINUITY AND ITS DEVELOPMENTAL VICISSITUDES—WHAT YOUNG PEOPLE HAVE TO SAY ABOUT THE PARADOX OF SAMENESS AND CHANGE

> The concept of a personal self necessarily assumes the ability to model the future as well as the past into some correlated scene.
> G. M. Edelman, *Bright Air, Brilliant Fire*

The present chapter is given over to two tasks. The first of these is methodological and involves laying out the specific ways and means that we followed in collecting and scoring and organizing the first wave of our data collection. Second, we will report on two early pilot studies in which at least some of these methods and procedures were put to the test in a normative sample of young people, with the aims of assessing the effectiveness of this research approach and of accumulating some initial evidence about the developing self-continuity warranting practices of culturally mainstream adolescents.

What complicates this otherwise straightforward descriptive enterprise is the length of time we have been at it. The research described in this and subsequent chapters unfolded in fits and starts, our ways of doing things evolved, and the young people whose thoughts about selfhood we have been most interested in changed in complexion over the course of our more than 10-year effort. In trying to be clear about all of this, we could have opted for a simple chronology, beginning with first things first and then serially rehearsing each of our changing ways of doing business, along with each new methodological refinement. Although some part of such a historical account is required if we are to avoid confusion, it seemed altogether better to begin instead with our current best thoughts about how to measure and score young people's ideas concerning their own or others' temporal persistence, and to only flash back to earlier accounting practices when necessary to clarify relevant details about our beginning and less practiced ways of proceeding. We first present an account of our current methods and procedures, followed by a descriptive account that explicates the range of distinctive ways the young people we worked with have tried to make sense of their own and others' self-continuity in time. In doing this, we lay out a detailed typology and associated coding scheme that represents our best efforts to capture the diversity and complexity of these participants' responses. We then present some summary findings that describe the relations between the self-continuity warranting practices of a group of culturally mainstream adolescents who differed in terms of their ages and levels of cognitive developmental maturity.

GENERAL METHODOLOGY: ASSESSMENT PROCEDURES AND MEASUREMENTS

The various methods and procedures that were employed fall naturally into two loose groupings. The first and largest is about our evolving efforts to develop measurement tools for getting at the self-continuity warranting practices of our respondents, as well as the coding schemes for characterizing those practices. Here, more needs to be said, and said more concretely, about our primary distinction between Essentialist and Narrative strategies, and about the changing procedural ways that we went about observing and scoring these practices.

Second, as we went about the business of inventing (largely from the ground up) various ways of indexing adolescent approaches to the problem of personal persistence, we were concerned that we might easily mistake Narrativity for Essentialism or for something else entirely simply because some of our respondents had greater verbal facility than others, or employed different vocabularies for describing selfhood and personhood, or were otherwise differently driven by their ethnic commitments and values. As checks on these several disruptive possibilities, a number of control measures were employed, which are previewed here and described in detail in chapter VI.

Using Pennebaker's *Linguistic Inquiry and Word Count* (LIWC) text analysis program and strategy (Pennebaker & King, 1999), we calculated some 74 language and text dimensions descriptive of the interview protocols of our respondents. A version of the widely employed Twenty Statements Test (Kuhn & McPartland, 1954) was administered to a subset of our participants as a way of exploring possible group differences in their conceptual resources for talking about selfhood, and a battery of measures of ethnic identification was also administered.

Additionally, details about our various groups of respondents need to be provided. In just one of the several studies to be reported, for example, we interviewed and otherwise assessed upward of 200 young respondents who varied by sex, age, Aboriginal status, and "place" along an urban-rural continuum. Some of the participants responded to all and others to only some of our measures. Again, some but not all of our young collaborators participated in a second follow-up session two years later. The particulars of this longitudinal sample, along with those of everyone else who cooperated in this study sequence, are laid out in detail, as circumstance indicates, in chapters IV, V, and VI.

Of all of these details, the ones having to do with the shifting and age-graded ways that young people talk about their own and others' temporal persistence are the most unfamiliar, and so are spelled out below in greatest detail.

Essentialist and Narrative Self-Continuity Warrants

There was little guidance in either the available literature or in psychology's general set of methodological tools to directly resolve our assessment problem of measuring how young people generally succeed, but sometimes fail, in thinking about personal persistence. We quickly learned that it simply won't do to merely ask point-blank how a given adolescent warrants her conviction about self-continuity or justifies her beliefs concerning the "diachronic singleness" (Strawson, 1999) of others. Young people, not surprisingly, look at you rather strangely when you come at them in this head-on fashion. Nor is this measurement problem likely to be solved by simply giving in to the familiar impulse to invent yet another Likert-type scale or usual self-report inventory. This is true, not only because of general limitations inherent in such survey methods, but also because of procedural problems owed to what has become the cross-cultural nature of our own research agenda. Here are some of those central limitations and problems.

First, and quite apart from any questions that might arise out of anticipated differences between young persons of different ages or because some were reared in this culture as opposed to that, the very nature of our problem (young people's self-continuity warranting practices) militated against the possible use of simple self-report measures or paper-and-pencil rating scales. Our primary measurement difficulty arose from the fact that, in contrast to more usual attempts to get at some denotative dimension of "self-concept" or some evaluative attitude toward one's attributes or features—all important parts of the contemporary study of identity development—our target was altogether more action oriented or procedural. As Strawson (1999, p. 2) argued, those aspects of one's sense of self in which we are most interested—aspects that are closer to what William James (1910) described as matters having to do with "I," rather than "me," or what Blasi (1983) characterized as "the self as subject"—are likely situated below any level of plausible denotative, or semantic, or declarative, or abstract propositional knowledge, though still a part of our phenomenological experience (see Blasi & Milton, 1991). Consequently, it is, according to Fiske (2002), often "worse than useless" to rely on self-report instruments in an effort to get at more procedural aspects of the self. Such measures, he argued, are "likely to [yield] distorted, biased, and confabulated representations" (p. 85). Still, even if all this were not so—even if such measures were, in principle, just the procedure required—our difficulties would still not be over. As Fiske noted, even if rating or other direct enquiry procedures did work passably well in studies involving participants from a reasonably homogeneous single culture, they would still likely fail when cross-cultural comparisons are attempted. "There are," he argued, "profound cultural differences, [even] in the meaning of filling out forms, let alone in asking personal questions" (p. 81), differences that multiply all the more when such comparison cultures are different from our own.

To complicate things still further, many of the measurement difficulties just enumerated are not exclusive to Likert-like rating procedures, but potentially extend to any free-response procedure that similarly presumes the face-validity of young, culturally diverse people's semantic or declarative or episodic knowledge claims. All this is true for the reason that what reliably divides one age group or culture from the next is not typically to be found at the level of those values and attitudes readily accessed by rating or self-report procedures but, rather, in the implicit practices and competencies that are "marked by their procedurality" (Wildgen, 1994, p. 1), and that importantly divide this culture from that.

If, as is now broadly argued by contemporary anthropologists and social psychologists (Kitayama, 2002), culture (and, we would argue, strategies for thinking about selves in time) is in fact largely procedural and practice based, then the best way to highlight relevant cultural and even age-related differences is to somehow obligate members of the groups in question to simply *proceed*, while taking careful note of how they go about their usual ways of doing business and unobtrusively recording what Kitayama (2002) called their "on-line responses." According to this advice, there appear to be two general ways of approaching our problem in such a procedural fashion. One of these, strongly advocated by Fiske and other fieldwork-oriented anthropologists, effectively amounts to "going native" [sic] and restricting one's involvement to "observation and imitation" (Fiske, 2002, p. 85). On this account the researcher, who is viewed as the only trustworthy "criterion instrument," must live and learn by being socialized into the target culture in much the same way that, as children, local residents were themselves once socialized. What those who advocate this "total immersion" strategy fail to make clear, however, is how, after assimilating culture as "lived experience," such researchers manage to "rise above" the "distortions and confabulated representations" (Fiske, p. 85) that are said to disqualify the firsthand reports of rank and file members of the culture in question. If ethnographers can do it, why can't they?

Until this problem is satisfactorily resolved, the remaining "approved" alternative (Fiske, 2002) would appear to be the use of new and minimally obtrusive measurement strategies (Kitayama, 2002) that rely on so-called "scenario instruments," instruments that aim to put respondents through whatever procedural paces are required in order to allow us to see their distinctive developmentally or culturally specific strategies in action. Figuring out how best to act on all this good advice, without taking up residence in a different culture, became the methodological challenge confronting our own measurement efforts.

One final obstacle blocking our path in coming to some workable assessment procedure arose out of the fact that, although being personally persistent may well be an unremitting obligation on each of us, actively thinking about being personally persistent on a moment-by-moment basis likely is not. Rather, it seems reasonable to suppose that most of the time we are thinking about something else entirely, and only turn our attention to questions about our numerical identity or diachronic singleness when prompted to do so by perceived threats to our continuity, threats that are unlikely to be experienced as omnipresent but presumably wax and wane in response to more or less evident change in what are taken to be the relevant features of the self. Consequently, when time erodes the self so that it is marginally or even fundamentally different from what it once was, then questions about continuity, identity, and equivalence naturally arise (Turner, 1996). On this prospect, it seemed essential to devise some measurement strategy that could work to backlight any remarkable change to the self that might be sufficient to set in motion those available procedural means that serve to bridge any looming gaps in the plotline of one's persistent identity.

Measurement Strategy

Given that adolescents are often notoriously short of declarative self-knowledge and often reluctant to lay bare whatever knowledge they do possess about themselves, anything resembling a frontal attack on their beliefs about their own numerical identity seemed doomed from the start. The alternative measurement strategy that we eventually hit upon after numerous false starts was one of subtle co-optation and entrapment, and generally involved attempts to make our own guiding question about possible criteria for warranting personal sameness a question that our young research participants took over as their own. We worked to accomplish this not so much by attempting to win their hearts but by delicately mouse-trapping their minds.

Step one in our three-step procedure consisted of soliciting confessions about our informants routine commitment to the idea that they, like others, have durable identities. Perhaps because young people are so commonly driven by what Elkind (1967, p. 1028) called "age dynamisms" (that is, by their wish to put some comfortable distance between themselves and their own more juvenile past), it matters a great deal just how one goes about putting this question. Still, as Gelman (1999), Keil (1989), Medin (1989), and many others have shown, most young people strongly subscribe to the idea that they are persistently themselves, and are generally happy to say so. With this much carefully established, our general practice was then, in step two, to press our research participants to describe themselves, first in the present, and then (depending on their age) at a second point 5 or 10 years earlier. In doing all of this we urged and prompted them to supply as many descriptive details as they could. With these two sets of "now" and "then" descriptions in hand, we went on to carefully draw out as many points of difference as were available, in an effort to emphasize how distinctive our participants' past and present accounts of themselves actually were.

With these two halves of a pending contradiction clearly laid out before them, we then (in step three) went straight for the seeming paradox by asking our interviewees how they could reconcile their previously stated conviction about their own persistence in the face of the clear evidence that they themselves had offered of typically dramatic personal change. In almost every instance this proved to be good enough. That is, most participants regarded themselves as having been brought up short, and in need of offering some (to them) believable set of reasons as to how their own apparently discordant claims for personal persistence and their assertions of personal change could and should be reconciled or otherwise bridged with good reasons. These accounts, which were for some short and for others several typed transcript pages long, became our primary source of data, and the basis on which the particpants' responses were ultimately characterized as reflecting either a Narrative or Essentialist self-continuity warranting strategy.

ASSESSING SELF AND OTHERS

At least two serious problems remained. One of these turned on the fact that talking publicly about one's self to a perfect stranger (typically two adult strangers: one interviewer and one recorder) is not something that most adolescents relish, and that reluctance is multiplied when (see chapter VI) such conversations take place across a cultural divide.

Problem number two grew out of the fact that our procedure, as so far described, only worked to access thoughts about the persistence of "self" and not "other." How serious a problem this limitation might be depends very much on one's research interests and on whether people ordinarily think about their own personal persistence, and that of others, in the same or different ways. Although this issue is of potential relevance whatever the age of the respondents, its importance naturally grows in studies that aim to tell a developmental, and even a cross-cultural, story. Do young informants think, for example, about their own persistence and that of their elders or persons from other cultures in the same or different ways? Is their self-continuity warranting strategy Narrative or Essentialist through and through, or do they mix and match their approach to this problem as circumstances demand? And what about possible differences in the levels of complexity or abstraction or formal adequacy of their answers? Do we employ more or less complicated ways of reasoning through the paradox of sameness and change when it comes to our own life? Does familiarity count for anything here, or does personal distance from the problem bring out our analytical best? Are problem one (attempting to shout across a cultural divide) and problem two (talking about the self vs. others) related?

Although answers to some, if not all, of these questions are forthcoming, the early answer to at least the last question on this list—whether the persistence of self and of other are related—was a definite "yes." Most respondents answered in the same way most of the time, whether they were being asked about continuities in their own life or in the lives of others. This finding emerged early in our initial pilot efforts and offered a potential way around an initial reluctance on the part of many of our respondents to openly talk about themselves. That is, as our work initially unfolded, it quickly became apparent that approaching most young people with a long list of personal questions about the particulars of their own identity was no way to begin; consequently, for procedural reasons, if no other, we found ourselves driven to search out a way of posing similar questions about continuities in the lives of others—others who we strategically chose to ask about first.

Whereas asking about the personal persistence of others was judged necessary for all of the conceptual and strategic reasons just outlined, a moment's reflection makes it obvious that this cannot be done easily. Obviously, different informants know different people, some of whom are believed to have changed a lot and others very little. Where is one to find proper target cases whose circumstances are commonly understood and whose lives are jointly known to be sufficiently kaleidoscopic as to put to a serious test one's abilities to search out grounds for persistence in the face of change? The right answer, we determined, is in literature.

Stories of Character Development

What we gradually came to see as the not-so-obvious solution to our measurement problem—the problem of finding appropriate "others" whose personal persistence is called into doubt by familiar circumstance—was that certain literary genres are self-consciously crafted to be about just this problem. In particular, stories of character development, or so-called *Bildungsromane* (Kontje, 1993), are built to be about lives in transition, and, if they are good, to at least hold the potential of persuading the reader that they are stories about one and the same person from beginning to end. In order to qualify as bona fide stories of character development, or otherwise meet what has come to be the gold-standard for successful modern literature, their authors need to have crafted a credible case that the hero or heroine, despite starting out one way and ending up remarkably different, still qualifies as a singular person whose transformations and continuities are both believable. In all of this there was the germ of a solution to our measurement dilemma. All we needed to do was to persuade more than 400 adolescents of different ages and cultures to read some number of the great books of Western literature and to attempt an account of how, for example, Ebenezer Scrooge managed to qualify as one and the same, admittedly much changed, person over the course of one fate-filled Christmas night, or how Jean Valjean managed to work his way from being a galley slave to village *patron* without becoming a different person along the way. Fortunately, not all of that reading is necessary thanks to the miracle or travesty (depending on one's tastes) of *Classic Comic Books*. These comics reduce classic works of literature to several dozen densely illustrated and easily digested pages. With a set of these in hand our task became much more manageable. Adolescents could be persuaded to (a) read still further abbreviated versions of these "classics," (b) comment on what such story characters were like at the beginning and end of their stories, and (c) be struck by the transformations that occurred in the characters' lives. Most important of all, the adolescents could be engaged in serious discussion (discussions of the same sort that they were later led into about themselves) concerning the grounds on which they judged a comic book character to be one and the same person even after undergoing significant change.

Personal-Persistence Assessment Procedures

All of the above was, in fact, precisely what we initially asked the young informants in our research to do. That is, they were all asked (a) to read (and simultaneously hear a narrated audio version of) at least one, and more typically two, such comics or pictured stories very much like the comics version and (b) to respond, in the context of a tightly structured interview, to a series of before and after questions about the continuity of the story characters. Then (c) they were asked a set of parallel questions about themselves and changes in their own life.

At various points in this program of research a number of variations on this theme were introduced. More than half of the 10- to 20-year-olds we interviewed read abbreviated versions of either or both Victor Hugo's *Les Miserables* and Charles Dickens' *A Christmas Carol* (most of which were in what we refer to later as the "Comic Book Condition"). As a check on the possibility that our results might be unduly influenced by the reading difficulties of some participants, the participants in our later studies watched a radically edited version of the classic (1951) Alistair Sims film based on Dickens' story. Although our so-called "Self-Interview" was always given last (for reasons already detailed), the order of stories presented and the media in which they were presented were carefully counterbalanced. Finally, because it struck us as unconscionable to attempt a cross-cultural study while relying more or less exclusively on story materials drawn from Western European literature, we succeeded in locating, with the assistance of experts on West Coast Aboriginal film and story forms, the picture-book version of a much-repeated First Nations story of character transformation (*The Bear Woman*) and a film produced by a team of Aboriginal cinematographers that roughly parallels the story of *A Christmas Carol* (which we edited down to a length comparable to that of our earlier abridgement). Again, we worked to control the numbers of our First Nations and culturally mainstream informants who were exposed to written and filmed versions of these Aboriginal and non-Aboriginal stories.

In short, our measurement tools for accessing young people's beliefs about their own and others' personal persistence eventually came to include (a) Classic Comic Book versions of Hugo's *Les Miserables* and Dickens' *A Christmas Carol*; (b) an illustrated Aboriginal story, *The Bear Woman*; (c) excerpted fragments from the Alistair Sims film version of the Dickens story, and a short film about changes in the life of an Aboriginal adolescent; and (d) a Self-Interview protocol to which all participants responded. With occasional exceptions that are noted elsewhere, all respondents in the several studies were first interviewed about changes in the lives of two of the story characters listed above, and then were asked similar questions about change and sameness in their own life. Whether participants first responded to illustrated or filmed stories or both was varied in systematic ways across the several studies. In every case the structured interview that followed the presentation of these materials was carefully standardized. This interview schedule, and the identically structured Self-Interview protocol, are both reproduced in the Appendix.

The respondents in all of the studies reported here were volunteers who signed informed consent agreements matching those already provided by their parent(s) or guardian(s), and (regardless of their level of participation) all were paid a nominal participation fee. All were accompanied to their individual interview by an adult member of their school, hospital, or Aboriginal Band. Two project staff members (one a First Nations coworker in the case of Aboriginal respondents) participated in each interview—one as an observer-recorder. All interviews were audiotape recorded, and typically lasted for 1 hour. With some (particularly the youngest) respondents these interviews were broken into two 30-minute sessions. As detailed later, some of the participants, depending on the study in which they were involved, also completed other questionnaires and paper-and-pencil assessment measures.

The details of these secondary measures will be introduced as the need arises, but here we provide a close accounting of the coding scheme that evolved across the course of our multiple studies. Not all parts of this resulting typology of alternative continuity warranting strategies were available at the very outset of our program of research. This is particularly the case with respect to those portions of our eventual coding scheme that have mostly to do with various Narrative solution strategies—response types that only fully emerged in countable numbers after we began including First Nations youth in our samples. For the sake of clarity, we detail below our current and best accounting of this categorizing scheme, and will work to make plain those earlier occasions on which all the scoring distinctions on which we subsequently came to rely were not yet available.

A Typology of Alternative Self-Continuity Warrants

Summed across the several studies we report, all of these assessment efforts resulted in some 500 pages of typed transcripts that required being coded (often multiply coded) in ways that are detailed in the following subsections. The part of these coding efforts that by now will sound at least somewhat familiar is the part having to do with deciding whether the continuity warranting practices employed by our informants generally qualified as being representative of what we term either an Essentialist track or a Narrative track. What we hope to capture by this particular choice of language is the fact that, even though our informants varied in age and general cognitive sophistication and consequently responded to our interview probes in more or less complex ways, it was still typically possible to reliably code their varied remarks as instances of either an overall Narrative or Essentialist trajectory or track. We prefer the term "track" to the more static and categorical sounding notion of "type" because it carries with it some of the connotations of forward developmental movement that we mean to emphasize.

What are still left obscured by these broad category judgments are all of the more or less sophisticated forms that these alternative continuity warranting strategies can and did take. Altogether, we succeeded in conceptually and empirically distinguishing five levels each of the Essentialist and Narrative accounts (see Table 1). The claim that we make about these parallel sets of levels is that together they form an ascending sequence of increasingly "adequate" ways of framing Essentialist or Narrative arguments. That is, each of the levels that together make up either the Narrative or Essentialist track represents response types marked

TABLE 1

Forms of Personal Persistence Warrants

Track I: Essentialist Selves as Enduring "Entities"	Track II: Narrative Selfhood within a "Relational" Framework
Level 1: Simple Inclusion Accounts	Level 1: Episodic Accounts
Level 2: Topological Accounts	Level 2: Picaresque Accounts
Level 3: Preformist Accounts	Level 3: Causal Accounts
Level 4: Frankly Essentialist Accounts	Level 4: Frankly Narrative Accounts
Level 5: Revisionist Accounts	Level 5: Interpretive Accounts

by the degree to which they make room for evidence of both sameness and change. Essentialist levels judged to be lower in these sequences, for example, either argued sameness at the expense of change or, in more or less heavy-handed ways, discounted or trivialized or bracketed change in ways intended to secure permanence on the cheap. What immediately follows is a more detailed accounting of this proposed and practiced scoring typology. This account begins, as our research began, with a detailing of the Essentialist track, and its associated five levels, all before turning to a parallel account of different levels within the Narrative track.

A TYPOLOGY OF ALTERNATIVE CONTINUITY WARRANTS

Track I: Essentialist Explanatory Frameworks

The five distinctive sorts of entity-based continuity warranting strategies that we have brought together under the broad banner of Essentialism, or Track I, have as their common denominator the fact that those who employed them all imagined it is possible vouchsafe personal persistence by identifying some aspect of self or other that stands apart from time, thereby justifying their minimizing the significance of personal changes recognized to be occurring elsewhere. When confronted with evidence of large-scale personal change, the first impulse of all of our respondents who had, in one way or another, taken an Essentialist turn was to identify something more enduring, something supposedly immune to the ravages of time. That is, they worked to define themselves and others in terms of some more or less abstract or substantive "entity" or "essence" (Barclay & Smith, 1990) that they understood to stand apart or hide out from time in ways that rendered those personal changes that do inevitably occur as somehow only partial, or merely presentational, or otherwise trivial.

The five progressive levels of Essentialist forms of argumentation that emerged from our analysis are labeled Simple Inclusion, Topological, Preformist, Frankly Essentialist, and Revisionist continuity warranting practices. We describe them in turn.

Level 1: Simple Inclusion Arguments

The least elaborate of these Essentialist accounting strategies, the Simple Inclusion Arguments, are predicated on an "add on" picture of personhood according to which each of us is imagined to be something analogous to what Lacan (1968, p. 599) called a *"corps morcele"* or "body in parts," some loosely federated additive assemblage of juxtaposed autobiographical bits and pieces that are haphazardly collaged on and can be just as easily sloughed off. When compelling evidence of personal change was highlighted, respondents who used this strategy effectively changed the subject by redirecting attention toward something else about themselves or others that was, at least for the moment, more change resistant. The individual elements of this building bricolage were generally seen to come and go without remarkable consequence, or without seriously calling into question issues of personal persistence, at least as long as the remnant bits and pieces still available included at least one discrete atomic fact that stubbornly remained and could still be pointed to as the guarantor of one's diachronic singularity.

Although evidently only minimally committed to the notion that claims on behalf of personal persistence require serious backing, whatever part of this obligation respondents pursuing Level 1 response strategies experienced was apparently seen by them to be easily satisfied by whatever leap-to-mind, concrete, often physicalistic feature of the self appeared to have most successfully withstood the ravages of time. More particularly, those of our respondents who were scored at this Simple Inclusion level were quick to grant that they or others had changed in all of the ways that they themselves had listed, but went on to happily rest their case for continuity on the persistence of names, addresses, the stray strawberry birthmark, or whatever random signature feature of their identity came most readily to mind.

What is obviously wrong with this simplest of Essentialist strategies is that it fails to seriously engage the permanence-change dialectic, and adopts instead a less articulated, divide-and-conquer solution strategy that centers exclusively on sameness, while simply ignoring change. Worse still, although readily available emblematic badges of personal persistence (one's fingerprints, for example) do ordinarily manage to stand somewhat apart from time, they are, nevertheless, typically rather poor at passing what philosophers (and life) call "survival tests" (i.e., If you are still you only because your fingerprints endure, what would happen if your hands were cut off?). In short, such Simple Inclusion (Track I, Level 1) continuity warranting strategies can generally be made to work only by trivializing who or what it is that we take ourselves to be.

Examples. Respondents coded at this level ordinarily had little to say about change, and concentrated their attention almost exclusively on whatever ready-to-hand thing that, for the moment, seemed to be standing pat, including: "My name is the same." "I guess it is my DNA, it's always the same." "… the way he looks is the same … just his actions are different."

Still, not every version of such Simple Inclusion arguments is as "simple" as those just listed out. John Updike (1989) captures something of the special flavor of more grown-up instances of Level 1 Essentialist arguments in the following passage about an old puncture wound.

> In the palm of my right hand, in the meaty part below the index finger, exists a small dark dot, visible below the translucent skin, a dot that is I know the graphite remains of a stab with a freshly sharpened pencil that I accidentally gave myself in junior high school one day, hurrying between classes in the hall, a moment among countless forgotten moments that has this ineradicable memorial. I still remember how it hurt, and slightly bled—a slow dark drop of blood, round as a drop of mercury. I think of it often. (p. 213)

It is possible to be both literate and at Level 1, but more often, when more mature judgment is brought to bear on the problem of one's diachronic singleness, it results in responses (either Essentialist or Narrative responses) that are coded at higher levels. The more sophisticated forms of Essentialism that, with increasing age or cognitive complexity, commonly take the place of such Level 1 arguments still share in common a reliance on identifying some unchanging part on which claims for persistence are made to rest. What does ordinarily change is the level of abstraction or internality at which such structural claims are pitched, and in the amount of care and concern taken to explain away the relevance of those aspects of the self or other that do suffer evident change.

Level 2: Topological Accounts

The defining character of the second Essentialist-based group of continuity warranting strategies, *Topological* (I-2), is that they begin by rejecting as inadequate all simpler claims to the effect that the self is no more than some transient collection of arbitrary parts, and substitute a somewhat better organized *architecture* according to which the self is envisioned as a kind of empty surface structure not unlike one of those hollow polyhedronic desk calendars that presents a different plastic face or facet for each month, and that lends itself to being differently viewed from different vantages. Responses coded at this second Essentialist level were, therefore, the first to seriously flirted with the problems of sameness and change simultaneously, at least insofar as they evidenced some initial appreciation of the fact that their argument for self-persistence was undermined if evidence in favor of real, unadulterated change was simply allowed to stand. The tensions generated through this minimal engagement of the problem were quickly resolved, however, by discounting the "change" half of the sameness-change dialectic as being merely apparent or presentational, and insisting that, although one or another aspect of one's identity may well be thrown into temporary eclipse, real foundational change is impossible, amounting, when it seems to occur, to no more than what Shotter (1984) has called a spatial repositioning of parts. The continuity warranting practices that grow out of such topological conceptions of self do manage, then, to "solve" the problem of personal persistence, but only by discounting or otherwise writing off all real changes as matters of mere appearance.

Fundamental to this warranting strategy is the contention that, whatever others might hold up as evidence for the existence of some apparently novel aspect of the self, these were in fact already present from the beginning, although perhaps temporarily obscured (e.g., "It looks to you like I've changed, but that's just because you've never seen this side of me before"). The ideas that someone has an angel on one shoulder and a devil on the other or that some otherwise well-intentioned people are "mean drunks" are both familiar instances of these Level 2 forms of Essentialist reasoning. Considerably more mature expressions of this same polyhedronic approach can be found in Bakhtin's (1986) account of the "polyphonic" voices at work in the inner lives of Dostoevsky's characters, or in the "dialogical selves" described by Hermans, Kempen, and van Loon (1992).

Examples. Our own young informants often responded in ways that amounted to the same thing: "Scrooge will say 'I'm not that way any more ... maybe there's something that hasn't changed' ... maybe [he's] still angry and just keeps it to himself" or "Frank might have times when he gets depressed again and angry ... but then again, he could have his days when he just doesn't want to talk to anybody anymore ... like get back to the same old Frank ... that's what I think of people that change."

What sets these Level 2 Topological accounts apart from the continuity warrants offered by their Level 3 counterparts is their synchronic commitment to the idea that all of the diverse parts that make up a self are necessarily simultaneously present. By contrast, the Level 3 Preformist arguments to which we now turn allow for the possibility that some of one's enduring parts are, at times, merely nascent and waiting in the wings.

Level 3: Preformist Accounts

Third in this list of increasingly complex Essentialist solutions to the paradox of sameness within change is a class of, this time more temporally organized, Preformist models that make some modest provision for the workings of time. Such Track I, Level 3 (I-3) accounts of selves and their associated continuity warranting practices were variously maturational or "epigenetic" in character, and happily allowed for apparent novelty, as long as those changes involved the coming to fruition of some always present but previously obscured nascent aspect of the self, the eventual emergence of which was necessary and preordained. That is, although sameness and change were both recognized, the strategy adopted as a way out of what would otherwise be understood as a paradox was to view the self as possessing enduring attributes, attributes that, though not all equally evident at every developmental moment, are always immanent and merely waiting in the wings for their natural time of ascendancy, typically in accordance with some imagined prearranged ground plan. On this account, for example, the apparently novel aspects of one's character that often emerge during adolescence were understood (by the adolescents themselves) as being the analogue of related and more physical changes, such as the late emergence on one's "grown-up" teeth or one's secondary sexual characteristics. That is, respondents at this third Essentialist level continued to imagine that it is impossible to get more complex structures out of less complex structures. As such, Level 3 Essentialist accounts failed to allow for emergence of true novelty, instead regarding any seemingly new structures of the self as necessarily having already been present, at least in some nascent form, from the very beginning. Snapshots taken at different junctures along an individual's preordained life-course sometimes create what is, at best, the *false* impression that there is actually something really new under the sun. The appearance of novelty is an illusion suffered by those lacking a proper understanding of how life normally unfolds. Such epigenetic or maturational continuity-warranting strategies served, then, primarily to ward off such illusions by finding ways of winning the argument that, despite seeming evidence to the contrary, each and every important aspect of the self is and has always been, in some sense, present from the very beginning.

Examples. Level 3 Essentialist arguments included such comments as: "I know that I look like I am different, but I always had it in me to be just the way you see me right now" or "because everything she did, she could have done before—it was all there. The bear people just made her realize it was there. Like Valjean, Rhpisunt had Bear Woman in her all, all the time, but she needed somebody to help her see how to get it out" or "Monsieur Madeline was inside Valjean all along. It's just when he helped those people in that burning fire, he changed. Madeline came out and stayed out."

Whereas Level 3 Preformist accounts, like their Level 2 predecessors, did minimally succeed in dealing (dismissively) with novelty by gesturing more or less vaguely in the direction of regularities in the customary process of human growth and development, they lacked any really effective procedural means for counting some changes as being less important than others. That, in a nutshell, is the advantage achieved in responses scored as Essentialism, Level 4.

Level 4: Frankly Essentialist Accounts

Fourth in this list of increasingly more complex solutions to the problem of personal persistence is a class of warranting strategies that hinge on the introduction of something like a genotype-phenotype distinction—a division of labor that permits one to actively acknowledge and subsume change, rather than simply overlook or deny its existence. Committed to something like what Polkinghorne (1988) characterized as a "metaphysics of substance," according to which it is automatically assumed that foundational matters of great importance are always buried deep, such Level 4 Frank Essentialists are always tunneling into themselves and others, all in an effort to get past their changeable surface structure and down to the real essential heart of the matter, their unchanging core self. That is, persons who employed this strategy necessarily regarded the self as a hierarchically organized structure with a certain internality, the deeper lying foundational layers of which were taken to be more central to, and defining of, the true "essence" of one's unique nature. Given this hierarchical arrangement, change, or at least changes of a certain presumably superficial sort, can be written off as mere epiphenomena, while, beneath this transient phenotypic surface layer, there can still be imagined to remain at work some more subterranean core of essential sameness, some rock bottom of stubbornly persistent selfhood, capable of productively paraphrasing itself in endless surface variations.

Armed with this new procedural move, practitioners of such Level 4 (I-4) strategies were able to argue in favor of "real," if superficial, change, without also being required to abandon the possibility of personal persistence. This was accomplished by envisioning the deepest levels of the self as having a fixed foundational status, while more surface level attributes (mere window dressings) are free to vary. Given this distinction between those supposedly deeper-lying and definitive things that are thought to form the subterranean and productive but unchanging core of one's identity, and all of those endless concrete variations that make up the phenotypic surface structure of one's outward life, any change that can be made to fit within the second of these categories can be easily discounted as being merely superficial, and so really beside the point of personal persistence. In short, change was seen to occur only at the surface, while an essentialist, subterranean, genotypic core was imagined to remain unaltered.

Examples. Paradigmatic examples of such Level 4 Essentialist continuity warrants included such claims as: "I have always been competitive. When I was little I wanted to win races, now I want to get the best grades" or "Valjean was always trying to do the best he could. In the beginning people just didn't want him around because he looked like a bum. Once the priest had given him that silver he was able to get ahead."

Running through the things that are imagined to vary across different versions of such Essentialist accounting schemes was a kind of depth of processing dimension, expressive of the relative degree of abstraction in terms of which seemingly distinct past and present aspects of the self were imagined to be joined. Toward the shallow end of this continuum were, for example, relatively modest trait concepts such as "artistic" or "athletic" that serve to join the differences seen to arise when, for example, one's interests switch from the visual to the performing arts, or from swimming to field hockey. At increasingly subterranean levels one finds more disembodied notions such as "personality" or even (pulling out all the stops) something as lofty as an immaterial, featureless and immutable "soul."

By successfully getting both permanence and change inside the same problem space, Level 1-4 Essentialist accounts of this sort move importantly beyond the Simple Inclusion, Topological, and Preformist arguments outlined earlier. However otherwise successful in helping to finesse the paradox of sameness and change, there are potential costs to be paid for hiding away the enduring stuff and making what is publicly available little more than a cover story. Even staking one's hopes for persistence on anything as fickle as a "trait" can prove to be a risky investment. Given enough time, traits often change too. Souls, or something like them (which potentially solve the problem of personal persistence by claiming, among other things, to be both featureless and attributeless), are long on generality but short on interpersonal currency, and so work to promote various unstable dualistic assumptions about indwelling spirits or other "ghosts in the machine" (Barclay & Smith, 1990) decoupled from the practical concerns of daily life. Although change can scarcely catch you out if the essential you is entirely denuded of all of its potentially fickle features, this would-be escape hatch comes equipped with its own rather steep maintenance costs.

Level 5: Revisionist Accounts

Finally, and perhaps because people sometimes bridle at the fatalistic implications of having the presumptive core of their selfhood "given once and for all, complete and perfect, in an ultimate system of essences" (Schlesinger, 1977, p. 271), there exists at least one further form of Essentialist continuity warrants that we have labeled Level 5 Revisionist Accounts. What respondents who adopted this strategy seemed to appreciate was that winning the argument in favor of one's personal persistence at the cost of invoking an absolutely immutable soul or some die-cast personality structure was simply too high a price to pay for guaranteed protection against failing the test of diachronic singleness. Rather, they voiced a new disenchantment with persistence purchased at the price of even genotypic fixity, and worked to amend what were often their own earlier assumptions about enduring sameness by bracketing their present beliefs about core aspects of themselves as somehow provisional and "theorylike." They often did this by offering up various competing views about their own or others' personality or character, and by suggesting that either account was equally in the running for a truth in a way that was somehow beyond knowing. By such lights, claims about the basis of personal persistence and change are understood as something more akin to a "working hypothesis" than a brute fact of the matter literally uncovered by somehow turning the mind's eye back upon itself. As will be made clear in subsequent sections, such talk about revised or provisionalized conceptions of selfhood begin to cross over and are hard to distinguish from other more relational or Narrativelike conceptions of "reemplotment."

Examples. Given the relatively tender age of the young people who participated in the studies reported in this *Monograph*, instances of such Revisionist or Level 5 arguments were rather few. Still, responses of this sort were present in our data set, including answers of the following sort: "I am the ship that sails through the troubled waters of my life;" or "I feel like I understand 'me'—but I know things can happen and I'll have to see 'me' all different all over again."

Track II: "Narrative" Explanatory Frameworks

In contrast to their more Essentialist counterparts, those of our informants coded as relying on some Narrativelike accounting strategy were less quick to dismiss as irrelevant all of those parts of themselves and others that refused to remain the same. Instead they appeared much more ready to actually embrace change, and to harness or tame time by somehow serializing it or otherwise locking it into some maturational or cause-effect or plotlike relational structure that could successfully bind the different installments of their identity into some ordered "leading to" system of followable meanings. In short, for those who fell into the Narrative Track, questions about personal persistence were seen less as a challenge to ferret out those parts of the self that had successfully hidden out from time, and more as an invitation to find new ways of explaining how change from beginning to end takes place.

As hinted at above, respondents coded in this fashion also seemed generally less challenged by being directly confronted with the fact that they (or others) had changed dramatically across time, and when reminded of how differently they had described themselves and others "then" and "now," they often appeared puzzled as to why this was meant to count as some bone of contention. More often than not, they simply began again explaining how they were once this way and had later gone on to be some other way entirely, all without reneging for a moment on their insistence that, yes, they were, without personal doubt, relentlessly one and the same person. When finally clear about why this might be seen as a problem, they standardly brought out whatever sort of umbilical relations they were relying on all along to bridge such evident differences, relations they had tacitly assumed were already obvious. Like their Essentialist counterparts they were, however, not born into the world fully fledged, and so were not all equally clear about what they intended to use as glue to hold all of the diverse time-slices of their lives together. Nor were all of these brands of adhesive equally effective in keeping the story of their life from falling apart.

Again, in direct contrast to those of our respondents who proceeded in a more Essentialist fashion by trying to locate some entity-based island of sameness in an otherwise horizonless sea of personal differences, those who practice more Narrativelike strategies were further distinguished by the fact that they more or less rejected out of hand the possibility that there might exist some substantive something, some enduring architecturalized feature of the self, that successfully stands outside of time. Instead, these informants tended to rest their case for persistence on the claim that all of the various time-slices that make up a biography are somehow stitched together by the fact that they are meaningful and understandable parts of a common chronology or personal narrative. That is, instead of dismissing as irrelevant all of those parts of themselves that change, respondents of this second more Narrative sort dismissed nothing.

What distinguished the various Narrative efforts from one another was that not all of our respondents made an equally good job of the business of emplotting their lives, nor did they seem to have the same idea about what is entailed in making an account a real story. Consequently, it was again possible to distinguish what turned out to be *five* progressively different lines of such Narrative arguments, each of which had some counterpart in the wide literature on discourse-based or narrative approaches to the meaning of selfhood (e.g., Lightfoot, 1997; Rorty, 1976). Each of these alternative Narrative approaches to the problem of continuity takes as its starting point a different conception of the structure or architecture of the self, and makes different assumptions about the nature of the connections between the various episodes that collectively make a career out of someone's life story.

Level 1: Episodic Accounts

As is the case with those at each of the other Narrative levels summarized in these subsections, responses coded as being of this Level 1 (II-1) or Episodic sort generally concluded that the telling of some sort of story that was naturally shot through with time was necessary, if not sufficient, to guarantee personal persistence. That is, in contrast to the more Essentialist-based accounts of their less discursively oriented counterparts, a defining feature of this and all Narrative responses was that they each "take time seriously" (Schlesinger, 1977, p. 271), and otherwise reflected an understanding that selves are inescapably "beings in time" (Flanagan, 1996, p. 67). What does go on to set Level 1 Episodic accounts apart from other more complex Narrative strategies is that those who relied on them seemed to have missed E. M. Forster's (1927/1954, p. 51) admonition that just having a story "is not the same as [having] a plot." Rather, when laying out the putatively continuous bits and pieces of their own and others' lives, they seemed only to imagine, as Whitehead famously put it, that life is just "one damned thing after another" (Gallagher, 1998, p. 87). As such, they only minimally engaged the problem of continuity, and attempted to vouchsafe permanence by offering up a simple, add-on, chronological listing of the contingent events that, taken together, make up the episodic details of a passing life, a life without noticeable rhyme or reason.

Examples. "First Bear Woman dropped her berries, then the bears came. Then she was a prisoner ..." or "Because five years ago I was in the 7th grade, then we moved, later we moved back again. ..."

Such chain-link Episodic accounts differ from their Level 2 counterparts, to which we now turn, primarily because the young people who employed them apparently felt no compunction to lay any real claims about what, beyond the mere passing of time, connects one episode in a life to the next.

Level 2: Picaresque Accounts

In contrast to Level 1 Episodic accounts, responses scored as Level 2 (II-2) tended to represent real, if somewhat run-on, stories reminiscent of what Rorty (1976) and Lightfoot (1997) described as early Picaresque novels, or still earlier Medieval Romances, stories in which the episodes of one's own life (like the lives of Sir Lancelot or Don Quixote) are not so much actively "related" as arbitrarily strung together like so many beads on a string, *sans* legitimate plot or coherent changes of character. Although containing the germ of a plot, it is not much of a plot, and certainly doesn't contain much in the way of coherent character change. In fact, the whole point of such Medieval Romances and Picaresque tales is precisely to illustrate that knights are true and unwavering in their constancy. Similarly, some of our respondents told related stories about themselves, and they tended to return again and again to the theme that, adversity aside, they were, after all, relentlessly themselves. Respondents scored at this second level, then, like the heroes of the other stories on which they commented, tended to offer up what Rorty (1976) called "characters" or "figures," as opposed to something less transparent or predictable such as "persons" or "selves" or "individuals." What passed for a plot in these accounts was simply a listing of episodes in which the hero acted in ways that confirmed his true character. That is, they and others are understood to possess only a kind of "functional identity" (Rorty, 1976, p. 306), according to which one simply is what one does. Within such accounts circumstances change, but persons, so long as they are true to their nature, do not.

Examples. "Well, he would probably tell them the way he was and that he ... I don't know, just believed in his dream to become that leader ..." or "Even when I was real young I knew I wanted to be a doctor. You could just say that everything is related to that."

Picaresque arguments, though they do run some thin narrative threads through the sequential episodes of lives, do so minimally and rarely in ways that support more fundamental change.

Level 3: Foundational Accounts

Respondents scored at the Foundational level (II-3) saw the present self as either (a) the inevitable *effect* of which one's ancestral past was the antecedent or determinant *cause* or (b) the natural outgrowth of a perfectly predictable process of maturation. In contrast to representatives of Level II-2 Picaresque forms of Narrative self-understanding, subjects categorized at Level II-3 understood themselves and others to have actually discovered a sort of directionality or canalized "plot" in the form of such maturational or cause-and-effect sequences, sequences that gave coherence and meaning to what were acknowledged to be real changes in their lives. The defining feature of this Foundational approach, then, was found in the fact that the threads that stitch together the fabric of past and present lives were always understood to be fully determinate, such that the new person one has become is taken to be the inevitable consequence of antecedent causal events that set life on its unwavering, and therefore fatalistic, course. Here, self-awareness was characterized by a kind of nostalgia, or backward-looking sense, in which one's life is given Narrative meaning by tracing back some maturational/cause-and-effect sequence. In these cases, permanence was understood to be only apparent or epiphenomenal, and the result of a tautological argument in which one claims that "I'm always what I've been caused/led to be." All of this needs to be understood as an advance over still simpler Episodic or Picaresque accounts, which lacked this more diachronic, or "leading to," dimension. At the same time, however, responses of this Level 3 sort were unremittingly fatalistic, and trapped by their own determining past. Present life was viewed as only the passively suffered effect of which one's earlier life was the antecedent mechanical cause (Bunge, 1963).

Examples. "I'd say [Scrooge] had no choice but to turn into a better man because he didn't want to turn out like his friend ..." or "It's because the Bear People caught her and wouldn't let her go. She had to change, and couldn't change back."

The cause-effect sequences on which Level 3 Foundational accounts rest were generally contingent and arbitrary, and so lacked the dimensions of meaning and authenticity (Lightfoot, 1997) of later levels.

Level 4: Frankly Narrativist Accounts

What distinguished the responses scored at Level 4 from their counterparts at Level II-3 was not so much their "leading-to" or past-to-present orientation, which they both shared, as the fact that their whole understanding of such determinate relations appeared to have become somehow more liberalized. Available evidence suggests that this happened in one or both of two ways. First, respondents who operated at this level better understood that the causal effects of past circumstances were not confined within one body or one consciousness, but radiated out centrifugally to include the activities of others, including, for example, one's parents and teachers and others whose lives intermingle with one's own. At the same time, the respondents coded at Level 4 viewed themselves less as pawns of circumstance, or what Bandura (1986, p. 12) called simple "mechanical conveyors of animating environmental forces," and more like what Lakoff and Johnson (1999) called "embodied agents," who shared responsibility for the way that things went in their lives. Taken together, these centrifugal and centripetal forces acted to increasingly free them from the dead hand of a determining past, but obligated them still to consider the vectored forces at work in their lives, and to solve this differential equation by computing the conditions that they saw as dictating the broken-field course of their own and other's run at the future. They did this, in important part, by imagining, as Dennett (1978, 1987) and Flanagan (1996) have suggested, that the self works as a desubstantialized "narrative center of gravity" at work in one's own life, a narrative with a plot that one is obliged to "discover" if proper sense is to be made of what has and will happen. Consequently, this effort to grasp and explicate the hidden plotline assumed to be running through their lives was always a work in progress, and these respondents' accounts of themselves often began with some version of "I used to think that X, but given Y, I now realize that Z." In short, Level 4 respondents regularly saw the path of self-"discovery" as marked by multiple missteps and miscalculations that needed to be corrected if they were to properly duke out what is up with them.

Examples. "[Life] is just like reading a book and not liking it, ya know? Like if there's a change or ... if you skipped a couple of pages ... you continue reading it and you find [how] it turns out ... if you read on and realize what type of person [he is], like if he changed and if he didn't" or " okay I'll tell you something ... why he's the same is ... like you can't be ... you couldn't do this like in two days ... but (only) through a lifetime.... [Frank] mentioned that he was going to take a first step and that step was in a new direction and in a new life...." or "I used to be quiet and stuff ... but I had a change ... I just realized that ... okay ... I don't know how to explain it. ... I guess it would be a shock to others. It is not as much of a shock to me because I know my life ... and if they want to know out of curiosity, they could ask me ... and I could tell them."

What was generally missing from such frankly Narrativist accounts was any sense that, even given adequate resources, it may have still remained impossible to ever come to the true and hidden plotline of one's life, or, more to the point, that such "plots" were themselves a human construction.

Level 5: Interpretive Accounts

Narrative continuity warrants scored at this Interpretive level (Level II-5) were principally differentiated from other less "provisionalized" antecedent forms by the emphasis that respondents coded into this scoring category managed to place on their own and others' active roles in interpretively constructing whatever order was ascribed to the temporarily sequenced events of life. In particular, what largely set such arguments apart from those sorted as Level II-4 was their emphasis on the fact that the plot now imagined to best characterize the unfolding events of their lives was not some preordained drift in the course of their affairs that needed to be discovered, but, rather, merely represented their current best approximation of an imagined pattern seen to lend their autobiography some followable, if provisional, interpretive meaning. That is, in unrecognized concert with contributors to contemporary discourse theory (e.g., Holland, 1997), such respondents did not view their current efforts to emplot their own lives as the discovery of some guiding principle that could hardly have been otherwise, but instead regarded their own efforts at meaning making as only the latest in a perhaps endless series of attempts to interpretively reread the past in light of the present (Polkinghorne, 1988). In other words, because such informants responded in ways that signaled an awareness that the story of their life must necessarily include, among other things, what they now judged to be earlier failed attempts at emplotment, they typically evidenced a certain skepticism about the future prospects of what they presently took to be true about themselves (Ricoeur, 1983). Rather, the text of their life, "like any text, is 'naturally' seen to be open to multiple readings" (Derrida, 1978, p. 227). Faced with a potential cutting room floor covered in earlier drafts of their life story, such young people typically saw no alternative to effectively desubstantalize the job of scripting themselves and others, and so evidenced some recognition that, as Harré (1979) suggested, their only hope of finding real continuity in their lives was through their own ongoing efforts to make sense of them.

Examples. "It's like in your mind ... like Frank's past will always be with him, but he doesn't want his future to be the same ... what happened or what he did to his past ... like he will always have disrespect for that, but he can try to make up for it ... act on his past."

The Morphology of Personal Persistence at a Glance

In summary, this typology, with its two tracks (Essentialist and Narrative) and five associated levels, came to serve as the eventual scoring key against which the responses of the participants in our most recent studies were held up and classified. Although our earlier and previously published studies made use of somewhat less fine-grained distinctions, and, in particular, overlooked some of the levels that now compose the Narrative response track, these oversights are not sufficient to break the general thread of sameness that runs through all of these data. Because all respondents in the various studies reported here received both a track score and a level score for their responses to both the Self-Interview portion of our general assessment procedure and for at least one, and more regularly two, attempts to account for continuities in the lives of various film or storybook characters, as many as six different data points (three track and three level assignments) were available for most of our participants. This allowed for a variety of different orders of comparison, all of which are taken up in the studies that follow. More particularly, it was possible to determine whether participants responded in the same or different ways when considering their own and others' personal persistence, and whether the track or level of their responses varied as a function of the cultural content of the story materials employed or the media in which they were presented. To anticipate the results of all of these later comparisons, it generally proved to be the case that the large majority of participants tested in our most recent studies responded in indistinguishable ways (i.e., received the same track and level scores) regardless of whether they were commenting on self or other, and in ways seemingly immune to the cultural content (Native vs. non-Native) of the story materials employed or the media (comic book vs. film) used for their presentation (see chapter VI for details). In those cases in which not all of the measures collected were interchangeable, and when a single track or level score was required, participants were credited with the "highest" level obtained and were assigned the track most commonly or most adequately employed.

Data Quality and Scoring Reliability

Because both our assessment procedures and scoring criteria evolved during more than 10 years of data collection, no single set of numbers fully captures the quality of our data or the coherence and replicability of our coding efforts. What we take to be the best available window onto these measurement issues is provided by the largest and most recent of our completed studies, more fully reported in chapter VI. In this omnibus study, 175 Aboriginal and non-Aboriginal youth were posed a total of 554 opportunities to comment on their own or others' personal persistence. Of these, 513, or 92.6% were sufficiently clear and detailed to support our coding efforts. Here, then, as elsewhere in our extended sequence of studies, our testing materials and interview protocol proved to be sufficiently interesting and clear to produce useable evidence from the large majority of our young and culturally variable participants.

Of these 513 scoreable units, more than half (60%) were independently coded by two trained raters, one of whom was always blind to the sex, age, and cultural status of the respondents. With regard to the primary assignment of responses to Track (the Essentialist or the Narrative continuity warranting strategy), these raters achieved an 85% agreement rate. With reference to the potentially more variable matter of Level assignment, the overall agreement rate was 86% for all of the cases in which there was prior agreement on Track. These results, which are in close accord with other of our previously published findings summarized elsewhere in this *Monograph*, offer reasonable grounds for confidence that our novel measurement procedures and elaborate scoring typology did produce evidence that meets the accepted standards common in social science research.

Early Lines of Evidence

Before coming to the bulk of newer evidence to be presented in chapters V and VI, it will prove useful to briefly recap certain previously published findings—data that have in several cases been supplemented with the addition of new cases—that have served as pilot efforts and justificatory support for our ongoing work. Chapter IV revisits and supplements two studies by Ball and Chandler (1989) and Chandler and Ball (1990) that link absolute failures on the part of certain psychiatrically hospitalized adolescents to understand the basis for their own continuity in time to the presence of serious suicidal behaviors. Before coming to this more clinical account, however, the balance of the present chapter is given over to a brief synopsis of a still earlier set of studies (i.e., Chandler, Boyes, Ball, & Hala, 1986, 1987) that represent our beginning efforts to measure young people's beliefs about self-continuity and to set these findings in relation to age and more standardized measures of cognitive maturity.

Special attention deserves to be drawn to the fact that in neither of these earlier efforts is there any reference to what we have gone on to call Narrative solutions to the problem of personal persistence. With the benefit of hindsight, responsibility for this shortfall is now seen to belong, not only to our own initial culturally sanctioned biases—as Rorty (1987, p. 57) pointed out, Western "Judeo-Graeco-Roman-Christian-Renaissance-Enlightenment-Romanticist" culture is, first and foremost, an Essentialist culture—but to the fact that, as our recent data show, the large bulk (80+%) of culturally mainstream youth of the sort who filled up the ranks of our earlier study samples rely almost exclusively on Essentialist self-continuity warranting strategies. In short, Essentialism is quite common among the largely Caucasian, middle-class youth who found their way into our earliest studies. In retrospect, it would appear that the rare instances of responses that would now be confidently coded as Narrativelike were, at the time, simply overlooked or otherwise discarded as unscorable. Such scoring confusions no doubt becloud certain matters that we would prefer to have kept clear, but, as it turns out, there were simply too few of them to present any serious practical problems for our present purpose of rehearsing certain otherwise clear relations between young people's thoughts about personal persistence, on the one hand, and matters of age and cognitive development, on the other.

Pilot Study One: Age and Self-Continuity

The first of these initial studies was simply meant to pilot what was then a newly crafted measurement strategy and to explore the sorts of things that young people of different ages actually say in response to close questioning about the grounds for their beliefs about their own and others' personal persistence. An ancestral or first draft form of the typology, and the rudiments of the associated scoring criteria, described earlier in this chapter (or at least that half of it concerned with Essentialist continuity warranting strategies) was largely abducted from our reading of the tangent literature reviewed in chapter II and the emerging findings of this study. As more fully described in the earlier published study (Chandler et al., 1986), a total of 40 boys and 40 girls drawn in almost equal proportion and equal number from the first, third, fifth, seventh, tenth, and twelfth grades of a middle-income Canadian metropolitan public school system served as respondents. A sample of convenience made up of 15 male and female first- and second-year college students was added as a way of anchoring this age distribution.

Although the methods and procedures followed in interviewing the seventh, tenth, and twelfth graders were close approximations of those already described, the actual story materials that we used as prompts to discussions about personal persistence for the younger half of our sample were not. With the aim of offering story materials more in keeping with the abilities and interests of the first, third, and fifth graders, we provided, in the place of the more usual comic book versions of *A Christmas Carol* and *Les Miserables*, two other illustrated stories: one a scaled-down version of John Locke's classic tale about *The Prince and the Cobbler* who exchanged memories; and the second a synoptic version of *The Ugly Duckling*. The Self-Interview protocol was an early draft of that previously described, and was the same for all age groups. The entire interview procedure for the younger participants was approximately 30 minutes in length.

TABLE 2
TYPE OF PERSONAL PERSISTENCE WARRANT BY GRADE LEVEL

Continuity Warrant	Grade Level						
	Gr 1	Gr 3	Gr 5	Gr 7	Gr 10	Gr 12	Univ
Simple Inclusion	7	9	7	4	2	1	1
Essentialist	0	4	8	11	7	4	2
Best Explanation	0	0	0	0	6	10	12

Note.—χ^2 (12) = 71.318, $p < .001$; Kendall's tau b = .640, $p < .0001$. "Univ" = first- and second-year college students.

Scoring. Again, because of the early days in which this first study was conducted, the scoring procedures applied to this first round of interview protocols also followed a somewhat degraded form of those outlined in the first half of this chapter. Nevertheless, it was possible, for the purposes of this *Monograph*, to collapse these earlier data onto a rather more rough-hewn version of our current five-level Essentialist coding scheme. This was accomplished by (a) bracketing under the general rubric of *Simple Inclusion Arguments* our current Levels 1 and 2 (both of which operate by ignoring change); (b) collapsing, as related variants of *Essentialism*, responses that would now qualify as instances of our current Levels 3 and 4 (both of which acknowledge, but otherwise discount, change as being beside the point); and (c) labeling as "Best Explanation Arguments" responses that we would currently code as either Track I, Level 5, or Track II, Level 5. Each participant in this early study was assigned to one or the other of these three scoring categories on the basis of their best response to interviewers' questions about their own or others' personal persistence.

Putting to work the combinatorial scoring scheme just outlined as a means of regrouping our original (i.e., 1986) data, it is possible to reconstruct an 8 × 3 contingency table displaying our participants' responses to questions about personal persistence plotted by grade (see Table 2).

As can be seen from this table, it is clearly the case that, all other things being equal, growing older (or at least qualifying for a higher school-grade placement) does in fact co-vary with one's assigned place in our typology of alternative continuity warranting strategies; with older and better educated respondents most often assigned to increasingly higher levels in our abridged scoring scheme.

Pilot Study Two: Cognitive Competence and Self-Continuity

The second pilot study, though previously reported separately (Chandler et al., 1987), was part of a common assessment enterprise and involved a subset of 50 of the same third, fifth, seventh, and tenth graders who participated in Study One. In addition to completing the measures of identity development already described, members of this subgroup were also individually administered the Goldschmid-Bentler Conservation Assessment Task (1968), a standardized measure of "operativity" that allows the loose characterization of young persons as either preoperational, concrete operational, or formal operational thinkers. The aim of this study was to search out possible relations between cognitive and identity development without being forced to rely on age or grade as loose proxies for cognitive development. In light of the fact that the first study had already demonstrated a strong relation between grade level and reliance on one or another of the continuity warranting strategies outlined above, and in view of the different levels of abstraction presupposed by their use, there was every reason to suppose that general cognitive resources of the sort measured by the Goldschmid-Bentler would set necessary limits on the particular continuity warranting practices that these respondents could bring to bear on the problems posed by our Personal Persistence Interview.

For this reason, it was hypothesized that increasing cognitive competencies of the sort said by Piaget (1970) to define the consolidation of first concrete and then formal operational thought would accompany movement from the first to the third level of continuity warrants outlined. Reframed as a question, this amounted to asking whether (using, in this case, cross-sectional data) some relation could be anticipated to hold between "progress" through the three-level sequence of continuity warranting strategies outlined in pilot Study One, and movement from preoperational, through concrete operational, to formal operational modes of thought. More particularly, we also hoped to address the questions of (a) whether the sorts of reflective abstraction that Piaget (1970) took to be definitional of formal operational thought were or were not prerequisites for the kinds of interpretive or constructive epistemology implied by what we earlier called "Best Explanation Arguments" for personal persistence; (b) whether Essentialist warrants, with their evident reliance on at least first-order abstractions, would only be accessible to those with at least concrete operational competence; and (c) whether those characterized by only pre-operational competencies could hope to achieve anything more cognitively demanding than what we have called "Simple Inclusion Arguments."

In order to test these hypotheses, the results obtained from the administration of the Goldschmid-Bentler operativity task were cross-tabulated with each participant's assignment on his or her earlier uses of either a Simple Inclusion, Essentialist, or Best Explanation Self-Continuity warranting strategy (see Table 3).

TABLE 3

TYPE OF PERSONAL PERSISTENCE WARRANT BY LEVEL OF COGNITIVE COMPETENCE

	Level of Operativity		
Continuity Warrant	Preoperational	Concrete Operational	Formal Operational
Simple Inclusion	12	5	0
Essentialist	0	12	8
Best Explanation	0	0	10

Note.—χ^2 (4) = 44.6, $p < .001$; Kendall's tau b = .794, $p < .0001$, Cramér's V = 0.689.

As can be seen from inspection of the table, there is an evident and strong relation between these two sets of measures. Moreover, as hypothesized, no participant who scored at the preoperational level on the Goldschmid-Bentler employed more than Simple Inclusion grounds for warranting his own or others' continuity; and no concrete operational participants succeeded in responding to the Personal Persistence Interview by offering continuity warrants at the "Best Explanation" level, although more than half of those categorized as formal operational did adopt this strategy in reasoning about personal persistence in time.

To further press this analytic issue, we conducted a Prediction Analysis of Cross-Classifications. Prediction Analysis (Hildebrand, Lange, & Rosenthal, 1977; von Eye, 1997; von Eye & Brandtstädter, 1988) provides a method of estimating the statistical reliability of models of developmental change using cross-sectional data. In a Prediction Analysis, the cells in a table of cross-classifications are assigned either "hit" or "error" status according to their compatibility with the model of developmental change being tested. According to the model described above, cells 1, 2, 5, 6, and 9 in Table 3 would be considered "hits," whereas cells 3, 4, 7, and 8 would be considered "errors." The analysis determines the extent to which the number of obtained errors falls short of what could be expected if the profiles of individual subject's performance across the tasks were randomly distributed. Specifically, the analysis determines whether the value of the test statistic Δ significantly exceeds zero

$$\left(\Delta = \frac{\sum e - \sum o}{\sum e}\right),$$

where Σe = the number of expected errors and Σo = the number of obtained errors. In the case of this model, Δ = .609, z = 5.349, $p < .0001$.

Three broad conclusions can be drawn from an examination of the straightforward results of these two pilot studies. First, it was possible to seriously engage children as young as age 9 or 10 years in detailed discussions about their own and others personal persistence. Second, increasingly older groups of young persons did, as hypothesized, ordinarily grow more sophisticated in the ways they reasoned about matters of self-continuity. Finally, there were demonstrable and highly interpretable relations between young people's thoughts about personal persistence and key transition points in the general course of cognitive development.

CHAPTER SUMMARY

Chapters I and II were meant to make the case that the job of exploring how young people think about personal persistence and the paradox of sameness within change is important work, work that holds out the promise of advancing our understanding of key concerns about the course of identity development, and how it sometimes goes wrong. Chapter III, which has been all about how such matters might best be explored empirically, had as its goals the tasks of describing and advocating for a particular way of addressing this otherwise unsolved measurement problem, and of detailing how young people's responses to hard questions about their own and others' personal persistence might be conceptualized and scored. Finally, we have also offered some empirical evidence to support the common intuition that the way young people think about personal continuity in time is generally age-graded, and otherwise related to other familiar milestones in the usual course of cognitive development.

What we have not yet done, shy of a few introductory remarks, is describe how all of this is related to the problem of youth suicide, either inside or outside of Aboriginal communities. Providing these missing conceptual connections is the business of chapter IV, to which we now turn.

IV. SELF-CONTINUITY AND YOUTH SUICIDE

This chapter is about our original question two, concerning the hard to fathom fact that young people kill themselves, or attempt to kill themselves, in numbers that are all out of proportion to those in other age groups. Our original promissory note, laid out in chapter I, committed us to an exploration of the hypothesis that suicidal adolescents could be better understood if their self-destructive acts could be set in relation to their own struggles to warrant a sense of personal persistence in time. What follows is an attempt to fulfill that earlier promise.

Chapters I and II provided good reasons and authority for the claim that young people, along with more or less everyone else, are under an identity-preserving obligation to work out some viable conceptual means of successfully warranting their own personal persistence. The several findings reported in chapter III are supportive evidence for the proposition that rank-and-file young persons do ordinarily succeed in satisfying this obligation by adopting one or another of a finite set of age-graded, and more or less cognitively complex, continuity warranting strategies.

What we have not yet done, but mean to turn to now, is to run this argument in reverse by offering reasons and a line of empirical evidence in support of the contrary expectation that young persons who somehow lose the thread of their own and others' personal continuity in time will also behave in ways that show a lack of appropriate care and concern for their own future well-being. As a way of putting this possibility to the test we chose suicidal behavior as a stark demonstration of failed commitment to one's own future, and we proceeded to search out possible relations between failures to sustain a workable sense of diachronic continuity and the occurrence of serious suicide attempts.

We mean to move this case forward in two steps. The first section of this chapter is given over to constructing a conceptual bridge capable of carrying enough weight to move our discussion from its earlier focus on normative developmental matters—matters concerning the usual course of identity development—all the way to where our attention is recentered on developmental psychopathology in general and youth suicide in particular. Having made these necessary conceptual links, we then move on in the next part to a brief presentation of some of our previously published empirical work (Ball & Chandler, 1989; Chandler & Ball, 1990). We present old and new evidence that offers what we take to be compelling support of the claim that suicidal and nonsuicidal adolescents not only differ in their handling of the paradox of sameness within change, but that young people who seriously attempt to end their own life are also characterized by having, at least for the moment, utterly lost their ability to convince themselves and others that there is real persistence in their lives.

ON HOW EFFORTS TO WARRANT PERSONAL PERSISTENCE CAN GO WRONG

As with developmental processes more generally (Noam, Chandler, & Lalonde, 1995), a number of things can potentially go wrong with the train of public and private events that carries young people toward a more sophisticated or formally adequate understanding of the argumentative grounds on which their own and others' claims for personal persistence might rest. One particularly straightforward example of how the wheels of development might spectacularly come off is fixation or delay. That is, one can just go on getting older without also simultaneously getting better at juggling both halves of the standard sameness versus change antinomy, and so fail to arrive in some timely fashion at the new and progressively more age-appropriate ways of justifying personal persistence serially adopted by one's peers. In support of this possibility, ordinary experience, along with our own earlier data, does strongly suggest that there are more and less age appropriate and formally adequate ways of handling the problem of warranting personal persistence, and that failing to move along this trajectory in a developmentally timely way would be at least statistically anomalous and perhaps socially inappropriate. It would not seem particularly odd, for example, to hear 8- or 10-year-olds defend their convictions about self-continuity by pressing the point that they have always lived in the same house or are still called by the same name, but similar statements out of the mouths of young adults would obviously seem inappropriately childlike. Although such delays may well set one apart, and otherwise signal that all is not well in the arena of one's identity development, bringing up the rear in such a fashion is not the same as having no such identity-preserving strategy at all, and so would not obviously cost one all commitments to the future or necessarily predispose one to suicide.

Not all developmental disorders, however, can be laid off to matters of delay or fixation. Rather, psychopathology can sometimes be seen to emerge just because developmental processes continue. This is the case, for instance, in the research of Borst, Noam, and Bartok (1991) demonstrating that a group of hospitalized adolescents were actually at greater risk of suicide when at higher levels of ego development than at lower levels. Such youths, it was shown, became more internalized, leading to greater self-blame and depression—a train of events that eventually ended with elevated suicide risk. Higher stages of development, then, need not invariably be seen as more adaptive or beneficial.

A related case can be made for heightened risks associated with failed developmental transitions (Noam et al., 1995). That is, beyond the prospect of merely stumbling or falling into arrears, it is also possible that, in regularly moving from less to more adequate and age-appropriate ways of understanding one's own and others' personal persistence, some young people may lose their way, abandoning earlier and less mature ways of warranting their own self-continuity before coming to some next and more adequate way of solving the same problem. Such young people, lost (perhaps only temporarily) in the transition from one to another level of self-understanding, would, as we suggested in work reported earlier (Ball & Chandler, 1989), find themselves without any workable accounting system for thinking about personal persistence, and so are also without any special reason to be concerned about the well-being of the person they are en route to becoming. We propose that it is during just such indifferent transitional moments that young people are at special risk to reacting to adversity by putting their future selves in harm's way through various suicidal behaviors.

Imagine, for example, an earlier version of "you"—someone who, only weeks or months earlier, was still confident in her or his conviction that, just by hanging on to the same fingerprints or bit of embedded pencil lead, all matters of personal persistence could be kept comfortably in hand. Imagine further that, along the expectable way toward your own intellectual maturity, you came to the more enlightened view that fingerprints and pencil lead are hardly the right stuff out of which an identity worth having can be made, leaving you perhaps feeling somehow vaguely embarrassed about your own earlier and more childish thoughts.

Inside this familiar scenario, two prospects, two roads not yet taken, now potentially stretch out before you. You could, and evidently most young people do, rush through such an awkward transition moment and quickly adopt some different and formally more adequate way of thinking about selves in time, some more developmentally advanced and age-appropriate way of preserving your sense of personal persistence. Alternatively, you might become stymied—caught between stays—by rejecting older solution strategies before alternatives are yet comfortably in hand. There you sit, dismissive of your own earlier and now seemingly inadequate self-continuity solution strategies, all without a serious clue about an effective way of linking up your own past, present, and future. These doldrums, which potentially occur in the neighborhood of every developmental transition zone, tend, we have suggested (Noam et al., 1995), to be particularly dangerous places to languish in, especially when jobs like keeping track of one's self in time will not wait.

Now, if you are stuck in such a place and are otherwise lucky—that is, if nothing else bad happens during such awkward transitional moments—then, in due course, you will, in all likelihood, simply go on with the serious business of coming to the next in what will likely prove to be a whole series of alternative and hopefully more adequate ways of thinking about your life in time. *If*, by chance, you prove to be unlucky (e.g., if your best friend deserts you, or you are bullied, or get grounded, or fail one more pop-quiz, and if, "for the life of you," you don't feel a stake in or can't otherwise find some bond of kinship with the person you were until recently en route to becoming), *then*, bereft of the usual identity-preserving connections that keep all of us centered in moments of despair, you may suddenly find yourself at risk of throwing everything away, of putting yourself out of your current misery, all over events that, should you live to tell the tale, may later seem of little consequence.

If you remember ever having had such thoughts, it turns out that you are not alone. Available research (e.g., Ross, 1985; Rubenstein, Heeren, Housman, Rubin, & Stechler, 1988) suggests that, at one time or another, most young people harbor such thoughts of personal estrangement. According to some (e.g., Linehan, Goodstein, Nielsen, & Chiles, 1983), as many as 1 in 6 adults go on to report actually having taken matters still one step further by actively attempting suicide at some point in their formative years. Something of the same point is made by available mortality figures that show, for example, that adolescents are heavily overrepresented among the ranks of those who actually succeed in taking their own life (Burd, 1994). In Canada, where the research reported here was carried out, young people not only *attempt* to kill themselves at rates variously reported to range from 20 to 200 times higher than those characteristic of other age groups (British Columbia Vital Statistics, 2001), but the age-standardized mortality rate (ASMR) for completed youth suicide is regularly found to be as much as 5 to 20 times higher than comparable rates for adults (Burd, 1994). Even these alarming rates are said to be misleadingly low (Cohen, Davis, Miller, & Sheppard, 2002). Suicide is, for example, commonly said to run a close second behind automobile and other accidents as a killer of young people, but many of these so-called "accidents" are themselves often known or suspected to be suicides. The problem is more dramatic still in various "special populations." To get ahead of ourselves somewhat by anticipating evidence more central to the work reported in chapter V, comparable statistics concerning youth suicide rates among the province of British

Columbia's Status Indians (e.g., BC Vital Statistics, 2001) also show that the ASMR for suicide among Aboriginal youth is a startling 8.3 times higher for males and 20 times higher for females than the already alarming suicide rate for Aboriginals as a whole (Cooper, Corrado, Karlberg, & Pelletier Adams, 1992). The present point is to lay special stress on the increasingly obvious fact that the incidence of suicidal behaviors spikes dramatically during adolescence and early adulthood, and so constitutes one of those problems that literally cries out for a genuinely developmental explanation.

We are, of course, not alone in suggesting that suicide is somehow related to problems in dealing with time and futurity. Baumeister (1990), for example, in reviewing much of the earlier literature, reported that persons who exhibit self-destructive tendencies also commonly demonstrate a kind of temporal tunnel vision (Schneidman, 1985) or foreshortening of their sense of connectedness in time, which leaves them poorly prepared to plan for or even contemplate the future. Suicidal individuals also commonly exhibit serious distortions in their perceptions of elapsed time (Brockopp & Lester, 1970), often experiencing time as moving extremely slowly (Neuringer & Harris, 1974). As such, suicidal persons are frequently unable to envision a future that is different from their present (Yufit & Benzies, 1973), and whatever little of the future they can foresee they ordinarily experience as bleak and blocked (Melges & Weisz, 1971).

Baumeister (1990), among others, read all of this evidence and more as grist for a kind of psychodynamic interpretation according to which disruptions to one's sense of futurity are read as the *effect*, rather than the *cause*, of suicidal behaviors. Those contemplating suicide, Baumeister concluded, are literally trying to *stop* time. However true this may be, it leaves us interpretively empty-handed in two important ways. First, it simply puts off to another day the central question of why one might be committed to "stopping time" in the first place. One mystery is simply exchanged for another, without any evident residual gain in our understanding. Second, and in contrast to our own more developmentally oriented account, Baumeister's emphasis on unnamed subterranean causes offers no interpretive means of understanding the dramatically elevated suicide rate of adolescents. As several investigators have pointed out (e.g., Ennis, Barnes, & Spenser, 1985; Maris, 1981), although young people do kill or attempt to kill themselves in large and disproportionate numbers, those who survive rarely go on to become suicidal adults. Chronic suicidal tendencies are rare at any age, and if you survive your adolescence and young adulthood, then, everything else being equal, the chances that you will undertake to end your own life in the future actually drops precipitously. Given all of this, one might ask where all of the suicidal youth suddenly come from, and where they go, and why they come and go as quickly as they do? What seems needed, then, at the very least, is some sort of "process" rather than a frozen "trait" account if there is to be any hope of explaining youth suicide.

Among the candidate explanations fielded in an effort to account for the apparent spiking of suicidal behaviors in the teenage and early adult years are situational accounts that point to the special "storms and stresses" of adolescence (e.g., Campbell, 1981; Holden, 1986), as well as more biochemical accounts that draw attention to the upwelling of adolescent hormones (Pfeffer, 1986) and the associated distortions of mood and perceptions that often accompany these events (Shaffer, 1985). Although there is no reason to seriously doubt that such internal and external factors play some role, they nevertheless fall importantly short of adequate explanations. Stress, for example, is hardly the exclusive province of the young, and though depression is common at various ages, suicide remains rare at any age. What seems called for in addition to, if not in the place of, such limited accounts is an explanation that allocates serious attention to the signature psychological problems of this age period. Clearly, as Erikson (1968) has famously demonstrated, one of these is the problem of constructing a coherent and continuous sense of personal identity.

In contrast then to these other candidate possibilities, our own alternative explanation of the ups and downs of youth suicide is rooted in a self-consciously developmental account that puts special emphasis on the ordinarily changing ways in which young people draw on their changing problem-solving resources in an effort to resolve the problem of their own personal persistence in time. Our research has shown that they do this by moving, as their conceptual resources allow, through a sequence of as many as five alternative problem-solving strategies, each of which works to solve the sameness-plus-difference equation in its own distinctive way. The problem arises from the fact that, in the ordinary course of working through this critical aspect of identity development, young people naturally encounter as many as four transitional moments during which few resources may be available for solving the perennial problem of sameness within change. During such betwixt and between moments—moments when they have each of their feet on different rungs of their own developmental ladder, and just when they are most unsure of how to best commit their decision-making weight—neither their old nor their oncoming self-continuity warranting strategies may prove especially effective. As a consequence, their past and future prospects both risk collapsing back onto the same specious present where nothing matters except the momentary pain. We have proposed (Chandler, 1994; Noam et al., 1995) that at these dislocated, transitional moments the usual barriers against self-harm are lowered and the threat of suicide looms especially large.

Such an account is consistent with the familiar developmental claim (e.g., Nannis & Cowan, 1988; Piaget, 1970) that "stage" transitions are marked by awkward moments of disequilibrium, but avoids the "developmental reductionism" (Rogers & Kegan, 1990, p. 103) associated with mistakenly equating psychological disturbance with developmental delay. As Rogers and Kegan point out, "because the histories of many adolescents and adults who have psychiatric episodes are without prior psychopathological incident, if we hypothesize that the current episode is due to developmental failure in early childhood, we are left having to account for a long intervening period of quite normal or adaptive functioning" (p. 104). Similarly, locating special vulnerabilities to suicide in the transitional moments between workable self-continuity warranting strategies also strategically avoids the otherwise puzzling fact that, despite the astonishing frequency of suicidal ideation or actual attempts, chronic suicidal tendencies are apparently so rare (Ennis, Barnes, & Spenser, 1985; Maris, 1981).

On this account, then, what is most in need of explanation is not why some people seriously contemplate suicide, or even act out such thoughts, but why the rest of us do not. The answer we propose is that for most of us, most of the time, there is a "rub," there is some future possibility that death would put an end to, or some future prospect that we are not prepared to forgo. For these reasons, then, adolescents, for whom transformations of identity often come thick and fast, are at special risk of at least temporarily losing the continuity-preserving thread that guarantees them a sufficient personal stake in the future, a stake capable of insulating them against self-harm.

The still open question, of course, is just how we ought to undertake a real test of the merits of this otherwise unexamined explanation of adolescent suicide. Our group has so far undertaken to find answers to this question by proceeding along two different research fronts. One of these looks at the problem of youth suicide at the level of whole communities (in this case, Aboriginal and non-Aboriginal communities). These epidemiological efforts are described in chapter V. The other research front, which makes up the balance of the present chapter, retains our present individual focus, and concerns our earlier attempts to directly contrast the self-continuity warranting practices of groups of suicidal and nonsuicidal adolescents (Ball & Chandler, 1989; Chandler & Ball, 1990).

STUDY THREE: ATTEMPTED SUICIDE AND SELF-CONTINUITY

Our working hypothesis in this study was that suicidal behaviors, especially among young persons, can be at least partially understood by viewing them as the unwanted byproduct of failed attempts to secure some identity-preserving bridge linking one's past, present, and future. Because adolescents are living through a period of dramatic developmental changes, and because their age-graded ways of accounting for their own personal persistence in the face of such changes are also in almost continuous transition, they are at heightened risk of temporarily losing their grip on precisely those self-continuity warranting practices that allow them to sustain a commitment to their own future well-being. On this account we hypothesized that young people who are actively suicidal are just those who have stumbled at one or another of these transitional moments and are, consequently, at least temporarily bereft of any serviceable self-continuity warranting strategy in ways that their nonsuicidal counterparts are not. The balance of the present chapter provides backing for this working hypothesis.

As matters lay in our program of research at the time the studies to be revisited here (Ball & Chandler, 1989; Chandler & Ball, 1990) were actually undertaken, the easy half of the proceeding joint propositional statement described above was already well in hand. That is, we had already interviewed more than 80 adolescents, none of whom were suicidal, and all of whom, without exception, had successfully mounted some more or less sophisticated argument as to why they and others went right on being one and the same person despite radical personal changes. That obviously left the really difficult-to-assemble second half of the argument regarding the testing of actively suicidal youth still missing. Given such a sample, what we expected to find was a new line of evidence that, in its simplest form, could be arrayed in a 2×2 contingency table that sorted more or less equal numbers of suicidal and nonsuicidal youth into those that did or did not have some (any) personally satisfactory way of warranting their persistence in time. In a perfect world, and to the extent that our guiding assumptions were in the running for truth, then everyone in this idealized picture would occupy only two of the diagonal cells of this matrix. That is, all of our nonsuicidal respondents would be coded as having some way (i.e., any one of the five serviceable Essentialist levels detailed earlier) of counting themselves as personally persistent, and all of the suicidal participants would fail utterly, would be unable to offer any personally acceptable means of understanding why the person they once were, or were en route to becoming, qualified as numerically identical with the person they currently took themselves to be.

As we will shortly show, this idealized, picture-perfect set of theoretically expected values, and the real-world picture produced by testing what eventually became a total of 82 young persons, were remarkably alike.

Participants

The demographics of any group of suicidal adolescents and that of the young volunteers who participated in the earlier studies reported in chapter

III tended to be quite different. Therefore, any thought of pointing to already collected data as proof that nonsuicidal teenagers always have some more or less adequate way of reasoning about personal persistence had to be abandoned in favor of the more labor-intensive but reality-oriented job of matching each member of our eventual suicidal sample with a nonsuicidal counterpart of the same sex, age, and socioeconomic-status. The usual adolescent inpatients of public psychiatric wards are simply less advantaged than the typical public-school children we had already tested.

Our sample of suicidal adolescents, a subset of which was previously described by Ball and Chandler (1989) and Chandler and Ball (1990), was drawn from the Psychological Services Department of an inpatient psychiatric unit located within a general services hospital, a short-term diagnostic facility that typically housed young patients for up to one month. For a period of almost one year, all consecutive admissions to this facility between the ages of 12 and 18 years were screened and enrolled in our study if, in addition to the required permissions, they were judged to be of at least normal intelligence and free of significant brain damage. Thirty such young people, the bulk of whom were from lower middle-class families, formed the hospitalized sample initially reported in Ball and Chandler. Subsequently, an additional 13 hospitalized and 13 nonhospitalized participants were added to this sample.

Following an elaborate sorting procedure based on reviews of hospital records, and with the detailed assistance of the professional staff, all of these participants were assigned to either a high or low suicide risk group. Interestingly, the planned existence of a hospitalized and entirely nonsuicidal sample proved to be a fiction. The clinical record of only 1 of these 41 patients was found to be entirely free of any reference to possible suicidal thoughts, impulses, or actions. Nevertheless, 23 of the patients eventually enrolled in our study had made no known "serious" suicide attempts and were confidently judged to be "low risk." The remaining 18 had all made serious suicide attempts in the preceding 3 months and had been placed on "active suicide precautions" (i.e., no "sharps," belts, or laces; carefully timed nursing observations; etc.). Each of these 41 inpatients was then matched to a counterpart public school student of comparable age and socioeconomic status.

Taken together, these participant selection practices not only gave us our small but carefully chosen suicidal and nonhospitalized control participants, but a highly comparable sample of "low risk" or nonsuicidal hospitalized controls, whose presence in the study served as a guard against confusion concerning what it means to be both hospitalized and suicidal with merely being hospitalized for all and sundry other reasons.

Method

All of these hospitalized and nonhospitalized participants were administered a three-part interview procedure involving the presentation of comic book versions of *Les Miserables* and *A Christmas Carol*, followed by a version of our Personal Persistence Interview that was more or less identical to that described in chapter II. As a check on the possible relations between notions of personal persistence, suicidality, and depression, the hospitalized group also completed Beck's Hopelessness Scale (Beck, Weissman, Lester, & Trexler, 1974). School officials judged the administration of the Hopelessness Scale inappropriate for use with this "normal" sample. Following scoring procedures also outlined in Study Two, the transcripts of the interviews of all of our participants were scored and ultimately assigned a summary classification of (a) Essentialis or (b) Simple Inclusion or (c) None.

It is important to note that this third coding category was not used as a simple wastebasket for the protocols of participants who were unwilling or unable to respond. In the end, only one of the hospitalized participants failed to make a serious attempt to respond to our interview procedure and was coded as unscoreable. Rather, all of the troubled young people coded as having failed to provide personally acceptable solutions to the problem of personal persistence found the matter of their own and others' continuity in time a matter worthy of discussion, but ended by throwing up their hands, having failed to find what they judged to be an acceptable solution to the problem of persistence in the face of change. Their records were generally no less elaborate, and contained as many words as did those coded in other categories. Some of these participants responded by detailing what they had previously thought and had since come to reject as acceptable problem solutions (i.e., "I used to think that it was just because my name is the same"). In short, they tried, but came up empty-handed.

Results

Table 4 sets these findings in a 3×3 contingency table that cross-classifies suicide risk status by personal persistence warranting strategies. Several notable findings are evident from inspection of this table. First, like other rank-and-file young people, the 41 adolescents who eventually formed our nonhospitalized control group responded in diverse (and age-graded) ways to our Personal Persistence Interview. All of these participants (like their predecessors in the previous pilot studies) found some coherent way of linking up their own and others' past, present, and future lives. In every case save two, our hospitalized but nonsuicidal participants also succeeded in finding serviceable (albeit usually less complex) reasons as to why the person they had been, were now, and presumably would become,

TABLE 4

Type of Personal Persistence Warrant by Suicidal Status

Suicide Risk	None	Continuity Warrant	
		Less Complex (Levels 1 & 2)	More Complex (Levels 3, 4 & 5)
High	15 (83%)	1 (6%)	2 (11%)
Low	2 (9%)	18 (78%)	3 (13%)
Control	0 (0%)	15 (37%)	26 (63%)

Note.—$N = 82$, $\chi^2(4) = 71.71$, $p < .0005$, Cramér's $V = 0.661$.

all amounted to one and the same numerically identical individual. In telling contrast, 83% of our actively suicidal participants failed to find *any* way of understanding themselves and others as continuous in time. They sometimes remembered, but went on to actively discount, earlier thoughts they had had on the matter. They were not, however, as might have been anticipated, more depressed on Beck's Hopelessness measure ($r = -0.31$, $p > 0.06$). Rather, as far as we were able to determine with the information at our disposal, they simply distinguished themselves by being no longer able to find anything that they took to be acceptable grounds for imagining themselves as continuous in time.

All of this is significant. Not just statistically significant, but significant in larger clinical and theoretical ways. From a clinical perspective, it is not without diagnostic relevance that, although by most available psychometric measures suicidal and nonsuicidal patients are typically found to be indistinguishable, here better than 4 out of 5 of our hospitalized sample who failed to count themselves as personally persistent were also actively suicidal, but only 2 of 23 nonsuicidal patients would have been misclassified by applying these criteria. At a more theoretical level, our own earlier claim that "owning some sense of one's self as personally persistent in time is foundational to any conception of self worth having" was importantly bolstered by the fact that all those who lose the continuous thread of their lives also no longer wish to live them.

V. FROM SELF-CONTINUITY TO CULTURAL CONTINUITY—ABORIGINAL YOUTH SUICIDE

Adolescence, as we demonstrated in chapter IV, is a time of heightened risk to suicide because it is characterized by a string of transitional moments during which developmentally earlier strategies for preserving a sense of personal persistence are repeatedly discounted, sometimes before other more adequate alternatives are comfortably in place. It is at just such stymied developmental moments that the usual slings and arrows common to adolescent life can end up temporarily costing a subset of young people any reason to soldier on for the sake of a personal future they no longer count as their own. Although such an explanation may still fall importantly short of accounting for why certain young people end up losing the continuous thread of their lives and others do not, it does go some distance toward making more understandable why the incidence of suicidal behaviors is so otherwise inexplicably high during the adolescent years, a time that, at least when viewed in retrospect, is often seen to be especially alive with promise. What it also fails to provide, at least as our account has been developed so far, is any explanation for the fact that suicide rates also vary so dramatically from one setting or community or culture to another. As we now mean to show, youth suicide is largely unknown in certain communities but epidemic in others, and any satisfactory account of this fact must somehow make interpretable sense of this dramatic situational variability.

The obvious difficulty in attempting to fashion such an account is that doing so would require building an explanatory bridge of which one end is rooted in methodological individualism and the other is anchored in concepts and methods better suited to a different, more culturally based level of analysis. Although few social science concepts appear to have sufficient currency to permit their being cashed out in both of these interpretive contexts, we argue that "continuity" or "persistence" is one that does. That is, taking our lead from the work of Bandura (1986) on collective and personal efficacy and that of Smye (1990) and others (e.g.,

Rodin, 1986) on personal and collective measures of "control," we argue that the concept of "continuity" possesses a sufficient core of common meaning at both the individual and cultural levels of analysis to allow for a measure of conceptual movement back and forth across traditional disciplinary lines. It was thoughts such as these that motivated our efforts to explore possible ways in which the notion of "self-continuity" (which has already shown so much promise as a way of understanding the problem of youth suicide at the individual level) might also be made to work at the community or collective level. It was anticipated that communities that have worked successfully to promote a measure of "cultural continuity" linking their own traditional past and building collective future might also enjoy especially low levels of suicide among their youth. The present chapter is meant as a test of this proposition.

Before further unpacking this argument it will prove useful to take stock of what has so far been shown. Across the preceding chapters we have been establishing three main points. In chapters I and II we undertook to make the case that, on pain of otherwise lapsing into incoherence, all persons are obliged to find some conceptual means of solving the paradox of personal persistence. In chapter III we laid out a series of different ways in which this might be done in principle, and then marshaled evidence to make the case that culturally mainstream adolescents really do employ more or less complex versions of at least some of these alternative argumentative strategies, and they employ them in ways that form an expectable developmental sequence. In chapter IV we presented evidence that danger—life-threatening danger—abides in those failed transitional moments when one has already awkwardly abandoned as immature his or her own earlier self-continuity warranting strategies in advance of having yet come to some new and more adequate alternative. For such young people, caught as they are between stays, the future really is suspended and death really does become a live option. Having shown evidence in support of all of this, we now turn attention to the possibility that some part of an explanation for the alarmingly high rate of suicide known to characterize whole communities (in this case whole Aboriginal communities, in North America and elsewhere) may be traced to counterpart continuity problems that operate not exclusively at the individual level, but also at the cultural or community level.

Of course, alternative explanations for the dramatically elevated suicide rates known to occur for Aboriginal peoples as a whole are also available, and because no simple and sovereign solution will likely do (Carsten, 2000), what follows is not meant as exclusionary. Still, most of these alternatives either imagine that the real truth of the matter is somehow inherent to intrapsychic processes or they involve arguing that familiar sorts of acquired socioeconomic and psychological risk factors (inadequate income, education, housing, health care, etc.) that often cluster especially tightly around Native persons and Native communities are the real causes. In this view, simply being Native is enough to put one at special risk of suicide. But split alternatives concerning inherent versus acquired risk simply will not do. Such explanations either remain mute about a whole chorus of cultural matters that, at least since Durkheim (1897/1951), have been known to importantly influence the incidence of suicide viewed on an international scale, or, leaving the person entirely behind, they tell us something about how living well as opposed to badly is to be recommended but say next to nothing about why it is, for example, that young Aboriginal people, or those who live here rather than there, are at especially elevated risk.

Our own study agenda included an explicit plan to avoid as much as possible being drawn into one or the other of these split positions (Overton, 1998). Rather, the research we undertook and the evidence we now mean to present were undertaken as a test of the views that (a) continuity problems that work to undermine commitments to the future at all of these levels are jointly at work, not just in the lives of individual young persons but at the level of whole cultures and (b) those forces that promote or threaten *cultural* continuity are strongly associated with suicide risk across whole communities. Consequently, and in active pursuit of this plan, we now move from our individual level of analysis to an elevated epidemiological undertaking that has involved first collecting and now presenting evidence to test the view that strategies meant to preserve a sense of continuity in time—efforts that we have already shown to be related to youth suicides considered one at a time—also function at a higher level of abstraction, at the level of whole communities. In particular, we mean to press and test this point by calling attention to community level factors that are associated with suicide risk within whole subcultures, or even entire populations.

To succeed, we needed to accomplish several things. First, we needed to establish, as we did in the case of *self*-continuity, that we had some workable measures of *cultural* continuity that could be usefully applied to what turned out to be the 196 separate First Nations communities (bands), 29 tribal councils, and 16 distinct language groups that together characterize the Native cultures on the west coast of Canada, and that collectively formed the focus of our studies. Second, we needed to not only describe some study window and some practicable means of counting up all of the Aboriginal suicides that have occurred within it, but, more important, we needed to detail those sorting procedures that were followed in what proved to be a first-ever effort to examine suicide rates at the community level of individual Aboriginal bands or band councils. Finally, we needed to articulate those analytic procedures by means of which we undertook to relate variability in our more localized measures of cultural continuity to variable rates of youth suicide within particular Aboriginal communities, all in an effort to test the strength of the association we proposed also exists between *cultural* continuity and suicide risk.

Before coming to the particulars of the lives and deaths we studied, it is worth quickly rehearsing why matters of cultural continuity might be of special importance for many of North America's Aboriginal peoples, and why it has seemed to us that such population-based issues might be relevant in coming to a better understanding of Aboriginal youth suicide. As a way of making this perhaps obvious case, we mean to have already added to the chorus of voices that understand youth suicide to be intimately bound up with problems at the individual level of identity development in general, and problems of personal persistence in particular. Youth suicide, as we have shown, is widely taken to be a kind of coal-miner's canary, a relatively unambiguous outcome measure of potential use for all those concerned with better understanding how and when processes of identity development go terribly wrong. In addition, it seems that no one any longer has serious doubts that all of the familiar discourse, practices, concepts, means, and modalities of the self are deeply culturally contingent (Holland, 1997, p. 163), and so cannot be usefully understood without knowledge of their cultural diversity. Finally, Aboriginal cultures throughout the Americas have suffered through what are now centuries worth of what Carsten (2000) called programs of cultural "untraining" and spoliation that, for many, have both rendered their own traditional norms and values irrelevant (Clayer & Czechowicz, 1991) and severely truncated their notions of future "feasibility" (Cornell & Kalt, 2000), effectively dissolving what Freeman (1984) called the fabric of the self and culture. Given all of this, it hardly comes as a surprise that in Canada, for example, where our own research has been conducted, First Nations and other Aboriginal youth reportedly take their own lives at a rate higher than that of any other culturally identifiable group in the world (Kirmayer, 1994).

If finding ways of achieving a sense of personal persistence in the face of developmental change is a defining task of adolescent life, and if, as we have shown, failures to achieve a sense of continuity are strongly associated with the occurrence of suicidal behaviors, then, on the common assumption that cultural continuity is similarly a defining problem of contemporary Aboriginal life, there are equally strong reasons to anticipate that First Nations communities that are more successful in achieving a measure of continuity with their own cultural past and likely future will also manifest lower rates of youth suicide than communities that are less successful in their own efforts at cultural rehabilitation. This, at least, was the line of reasoning that led to what is reported here as "Study Four."

STUDY FOUR: CULTURAL CONTINUITY AND THE EPIDEMIOLOGY OF SUICIDE AMONG ABORIGINAL YOUTH

The data to which we now turn were gathered as early steps in what has now become a series of ongoing epidemiological studies. The full details of the first wave of this enterprise, covering suicide rates for the whole of the province in which we worked for the period 1987 through 1992 have been reported elsewhere (Chandler & Lalonde, 1998) and the interested reader is encouraged to seek the full details of our procedures from this previously published account. More recent lines of evidence covering the period ending in 2001 are reported here as well. What needs to be made clear in advance of summarizing these findings is how we went about characterizing the level of cultural continuity descriptive of each of the almost 200 Aboriginal bands that populate British Columbia.

If it were somehow possible to interview a whole culture, we could simply have asked, in a fashion analogous to the way we routinely asked adolescents, for a description of the culture at some point in the past, then for a current description, and proceeded to probe for some accounting of the apparent changes that had taken place over time. In the case of First Nations cultures in Canada, none of this has the ring of likely success. Little history is known about Aboriginal cultures prior to contact with Europeans. As part of a history that is shared with Aboriginal peoples across the Americas, Native communities in Pacific Canada were forcibly relocated, resources and lands were appropriated, and traditional ways of living were outlawed and ridiculed. In British Columbia, the Native communities' religious practices and local forms of government were criminalized, and children were systematically removed from their parents' care to be educated in residential schools. In an official recounting of some of this shameful history, the Government of Canada has admitted that these policies were "intended to remove Aboriginal people from their homelands, suppress Aboriginal nations and their governments, undermine Aboriginal cultures, [and] stifle Aboriginal identity" (Report of the Royal Commission on Aboriginal Peoples, 1996). By all accounts, these official policies were remarkably effective. Not surprisingly, then, the stark differences between past and current manifestations of Aboriginal culture make simple then-and-now comparisons meant to point up commonalties across time rather beside the point of contemporary First Nations life. What does matter—and matters deeply to First Nations people—are efforts (both backward referring and forward anticipating) to not only preserve, restore, and rehabilitate the remnants of their collective past, but to regain control of their own future and destiny. It was to these rebuilding efforts that we turned in our search for some measure of cultural continuity.

The kernel idea we have been pursuing is that much of what it means to preserve and promote Native culture is reflected in the degree to which First Nations have been attempting (and sometimes succeeding) to wrest control of their communities from government supervision. This focus on the devolution of various forms of government control into community hands may seem an overly politicized approach. Why not concentrate on things that are somehow more "cultural"—the prevalence of Aboriginal languages, or traditional methods of food provision, or rituals, or spiritual practices? First Nations are, of course, engaging in all of those practices as well, and are succeeding in passing on traditional ways to youth, but not in ways that easily lend themselves to epidemiological analysis. What we needed for our research was not some measure of what strands of traditional practice or knowledge had survived, but rather some set of marker variables that would reliably indicate how each of 196 distinct communities in British Columbia had fared in its struggles to resist the sustained history of acculturative practices that threaten its very cultural existence. Politicized or not, this reality is hardly of our own making. It is, however, the reality of the measurable things at our disposal.

We finally settled on a set of just six marker variables. Two of these index efforts on the part of communities to directly challenge federal and provincial governments for title to traditional lands and the right to self-governance by measuring the length of their history, and degree of success, in litigation and political action. Here we make a prima facie case that having been engaged in a long legal struggle for dominion over one's own place and person is as good a measure as one could want of efforts to regain control over cultural and communal life. Three other variables concern matters of control over provision of services that have been more recently begun slowly passing from government to local Bands and Band Councils. These include responsibility for education, healthcare, and police and fire services. Our final marker variable represents an attempt to more directly measure some aspect of cultural life. Without an effective means of comparing the importance of various cultural practices across these diverse nations, we opted instead to simply determine whether or not the communities in question had constructed a building devoted to cultural activities. In some communities, cultural activities take place in the local school gymnasium or in the basement of the local church. Without meaning to discount these make-do local solutions, we took it as a measure of collective cultural strength if a community had successfully managed to erect some permanent structure specifically designated for the preservation and promotion of culture.

What these marker variables may appear to lack in "cultural currency" when set against traditional language use or spirituality, they more than make up for in the breadth of their application. That is, even if we are unable to assess specific cultural practices within each community, we can count court documents and the number of Native-administered schools. Aided by mountains of government documentation, we did just that and were able to determine exactly where each of 196 communities stood on each of our chosen marker variables.

If these proxy measures of cultural continuity could tell us something about the will and the efforts of individual communities to regain control of these aspects of their cultural life, and if cultural continuity functions in the same manner at a community level as self-continuity does at the individual level, then suicide rates should vary as a function of their presence or absence. Therefore, our hypothesis was that in the case of each of our measures suicide rates would be lower in communities where the marker was present than in communities where it was absent. Given that suicide is a low incidence behavior, what we then needed was a population large enough and a window of time long enough to produce a data set adequate to the task of testing our hypothesis. We chose the whole of British Columbia and, in the first instance, a six-year time window. The details of our initial data collection methods are outlined below.

Methods

Suicide Data

We began by obtaining data on every recorded suicide in the province of British Columbia during the years 1987 through 1992. This data set included all of the information surrounding the death that the Office of the Chief Coroner of British Columbia is obliged to collect: age, gender, place of death, date of death, cause and means of death, and associated factors (alcohol, drug involvement, etc.). It must be acknowledged from the outset that this total almost certainly underestimates, perhaps by a very wide margin, the full number of suicides within a population. The total does not, for example, include deaths ruled as accidental, even when the driver in a single-occupant motor vehicle accident was known to be suicidal at the time of the "accident." One federal government agency pegs the number of accidental deaths that should be counted as suicides at one in four (Health Canada, 1991). This underestimation may be particularly problematic within the First Nations population which is known to experience substantially higher rates of accidental deaths.

The coroner's records also indicated whether or not the deceased was Native. This designation is not, however, as straightforward as one would hope. In addition to personally declaring oneself to be of aboriginal ancestry, the federal government maintains a registry of "Status Indians" and each First Nation maintains a Band membership list. Because these sources are occasionally at odds, when designating deaths as "Native" the coroner's office gathers further information from surviving family members, police, and other government agencies. Additional data provided by the federal Department of Indian and Northern Affairs allowed us to confirm First Nations membership and the location of the community to which the deceased belonged.

Population Estimates

Finding the appropriate population denominator to use in calculating yearly suicide rates for Native and non-Native groups also proved to be a challenge. Figures for the entire province were derived from federal census data that were then adjusted (for noncensus years) using provincial government population estimates. Because some First Nations do not participate in the national census, routinely available population figures for First Nations communities were difficult to verify. Fortunately, the timing of our study allowed us to take advantage of a multijurisdictional government effort to chart the health status of Aboriginal people that produced what are considered the most accurate estimates to date of the First Nations population of British Columbia (Burd, 1994).

Political Affiliations and Language Groups

As we noted earlier, suicides are rare. When summed over too brief a time span or across too small a population, anomalously high or low suicide rates can result. This statistical possibility was of special concern to us, given that many Native communities are small in size and remote in location. As a corrective, we chose three methods of categorizing communities into larger groupings. First, each band belongs to one of 29 Tribal Councils, which are cultural/political alliances that in most cases reflect a common history or language but in other cases are more political or economic. Suicide rates were calculated for each of these tribal councils. A second effort to avoid statistical anomalies involved grouping bands by traditional language. A total of 16 distinct linguistic families have been identified in British Columbia and (with expert advice) we were able to classify bands according to this metric. Suicide rates were again calculated for each language group. Finally, because of the size and geographic diversity of British Columbia, we also calculated rates separately for urban, rural, and remote communities.

Results

What we found, as has anyone else who has examined rates of suicide among aboriginal people (e.g., Kirmayer, 1994), was that the rate for Native

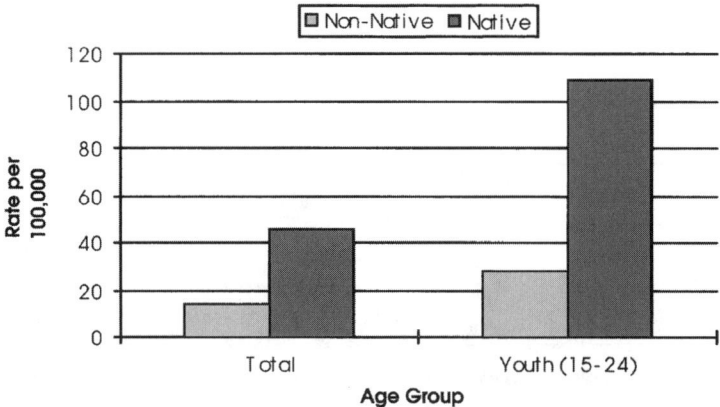

FIGURE 1.—Total suicide rates in British Columbia (1987–1992).

people was much higher (in this case more than three times higher) than it was for the total population. And, once again, we found that the suicide rate was higher for young persons than for any other age group (1.6 times higher). What was still surprising, however, was the fact that the rate for Native youths was nearly 5 times that of youths in general. As the data in Figure 1 clearly illustrate, words like "epidemic" seem apt.

Given that the Native population was (and remains) disproportionately young in comparison to the province as a whole, a set of age standardized mortality rates were calculated to compensate for differences in the age distribution of the two groups. These calculations estimate what the comparative rates would be if the two populations shared the same standard age distribution. In this case, the rates (now arrayed over the 6 years of the study) were statistically clearer, but yielded a similar picture (see Figure 2).

Variability in Suicide Rates

Our purpose was not simply to once again demonstrate that suicide is more frequent within the First Nations population. Rather, we were interested in variability in suicide rates across different First Nations communities. The logical next step, then, was to display the suicides rates for all 196 communities studied. Although rates calculated at that level are misleading, with the numbers ranging from 0 to more than 3,600 per 100,000, they did strongly suggest that simply being First Nations was not, in itself, a risk factor. Such data show, for example, that more than half of the bands studied (111 of 196) had *no* youth suicides during the study period. More telling were the rates derived when communities were aggregated in various ways to produce more stable estimates of risk. When communities

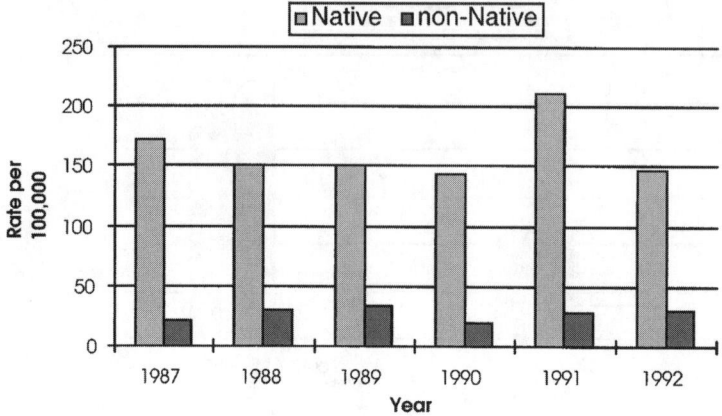

FIGURE 2.—Native and non-Native youth suicide rates (age-standardized mortality rates, 1987–1992).

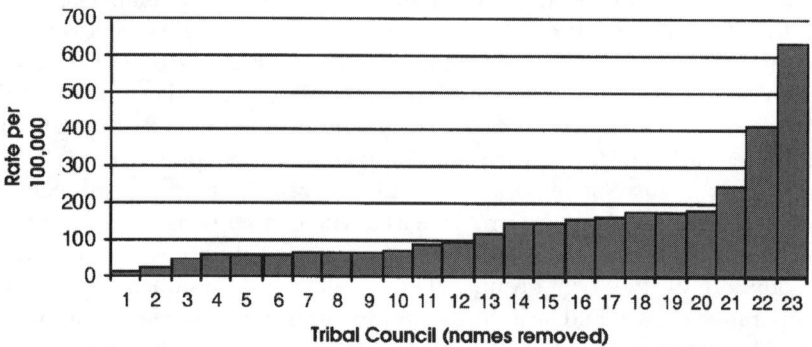

FIGURE 3.—Native youth suicide rate by tribal council.

were grouped together into tribal councils, variability remained but at a much reduced level. Six of the 29 tribal councils experienced no suicides during the study window. Among the 23 remaining councils, rates ranged from below the provincial average to as high as 633 per 100,000. These rates are displayed (with the names of the tribal councils removed) in Figure 3.

A similar picture emerged when rates were calculated for the 16 linguistic groups in the province. Five of these groups had youth suicide rates of zero; the others ranged upward to a high of more than 200 per 100,000 (see Figure 4).

As a check against two factors traditionally associated with variability in suicide rates, we also examined the effects of population density and geographic location. Density was measured by dividing the community population by the number of separate dwelling places. The correlation between youth suicide and this measure of crowding was essentially zero

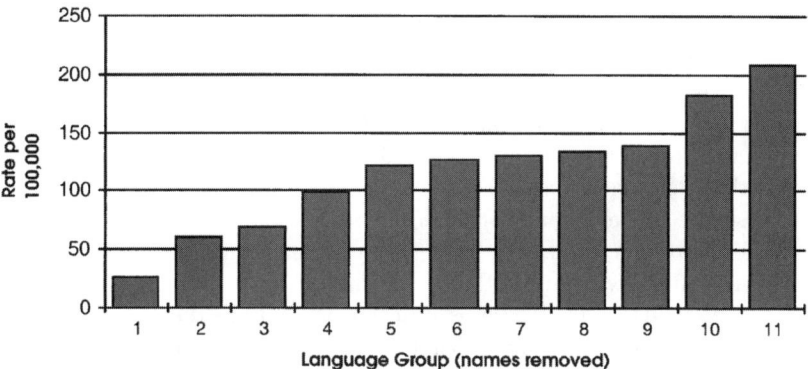

FIGURE 4.—Native youth suicide rate by language group.

($r = -0.05$). Similarly, categorizing bands by geographic location revealed a steady (but not significant) increase in rates from remote, to rural, to urban centers.

Measures of Cultural Continuity

What the data reported thus far indicated was not only that rates were higher in the Native than in the non-Native population but that wide variability existed in suicide rates observed within this collection of Native communities. Most had no recorded suicides, others had many. Dramatic variability would be expected given that nearly 200 small communities were scattered across the province. When examined by tribal council and by language group, however, where the population denominator was substantially larger, variability remained. We took this to mean that such variability was not just statistical noise but rather an invitation to search for some method of parsing variance that made room for some of the different approaches to cultural and communal life that characterized the groups under study. The set of cultural continuity marker variables described above would, we hypothesized, form just such a measure.

The final steps in our analysis of this data set involved gathering information about each of the communities and constructing a matrix in which each marker was judged to be either present or absent in the community such that suicide rates could be calculated for the set of communities that shared the same value on each marker. By way of reminder, our hypothesis was that the presence of each marker would be associated with a decrease in the youth suicide rate. Before reporting on the results, however, something more needs to be said about how each of these variables was measured.

71

1. *Land Claims.* In the early 1990s, a process for conducting treaty negotiations was instituted that was designed to include all First Nations as well as representatives of the federal and provincial governments. Because not all First Nations have continued to participate in this process (at the time of this writing, 125 of 197 bands remain at the treaty tables), and because participation does not necessarily reflect a history of struggle to secure title to traditional lands, we made use of both current and past efforts to divide bands with a long history of land claims actions from those whose efforts were initiated more recently.

2. *Self-Government.* Bands differed not only in the length of their history of land claims, but also in the degree of success they had achieved in their legal dealings with federal and provincial governments. One measure of this success was the establishment of recognized institutions of self-government that endow bands with a substantial degree of economic and political independence. Although more commonplace in the United States, such arrangements were relatively rare in western Canada.

3. *Education.* The funding of education in Native communities is an often complex set of arrangements between federal and provincial agencies and local school boards. The details are typically negotiated through local education agreements and vary widely from place to place. Although there are several ways of categorizing how children are educated in different communities, we elected to classify bands according to whether or not a majority of the students in the community attended a band-administered school.

4. *Police and Fire Protection Services.* Responsibility for police services outside of major urban centers is held by the Royal Canadian Mounted Police. Native communities, however, have (to varying degrees) been active in developing community-based programs for law enforcement on reserve lands. Similarly, fire protection services are often provided by neighboring non-Native communities in more urban areas and by a volunteer fire department in remote areas. In addition to contracting out for such services, many bands also maintain ownership of fire-fighting equipment. Our measure indexed the extent to which the community owned or controlled these services.

5. *Health Services.* As with many services to Native communities, control of healthcare provision is moving (at varying rates) into the hands of band and tribal councils. At the time of this study some bands had very little control over the delivery of health services and relied entirely on providers located outside the community or on temporary "fly-in" clinics; others had managed to secure permanent healthcare providers within the community. Because some communities were especially small and isolated, we chose to measure the level of control over the service rather than the type or location of the service itself.

6. *Cultural Facilities.* Using both information contained in government records and information obtained by contacting the band office in each of the communities, we assembled descriptions of all communal facilities located within each community. These same sources were used to determine whether or not one or more of these buildings was specifically designated or reserved for cultural activities.

When suicides were parsed by the presence or absence of these six marker variables, and suicide rates were recalculated, a consistent pattern appeared. In every case, the youth suicide rate was lower in communities that shared markers of cultural continuity (see Figure 5).

One measure of the "protective" effects of these markers is found in the fact that even the least dramatic difference in rates (police/fire) amounted to 24.7 fewer suicides per 100,000. We should stress that these rates were calculated over the entire provincial population and therefore constituted exact population parameters rather than sample estimates of suicide rates; inferential techniques to assess the strength of these findings were simply unnecessary. As a consequence, the reduction in relative risk associated with the presence of these markers can be listed without need of trailing statistics: self-government, 85%; land claims, 41%; education, 52%; health, 29%; cultural facilities, 23%; police/fire, 20%.

Though each of the markers was effective in its own right, we also examined their strength in combination. To do so, we merely summed the scores of each community and assigned each community a score ranging from 0–6 according to the total number of markers present in the

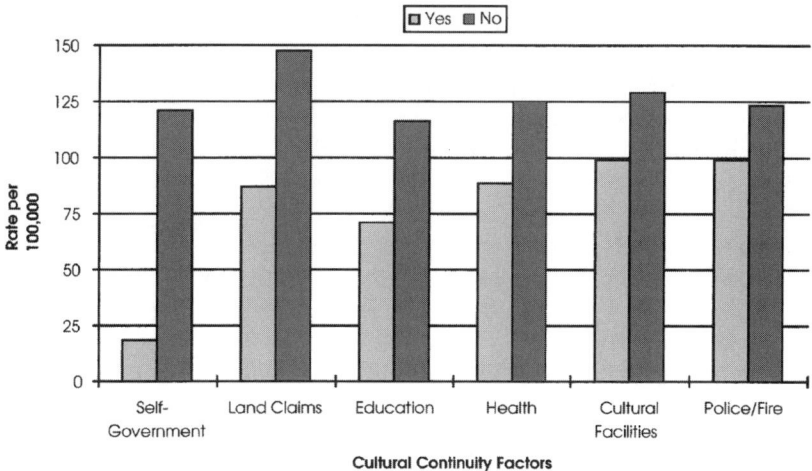

FIGURE 5.—Native youth suicide rates by cultural continuity factors.

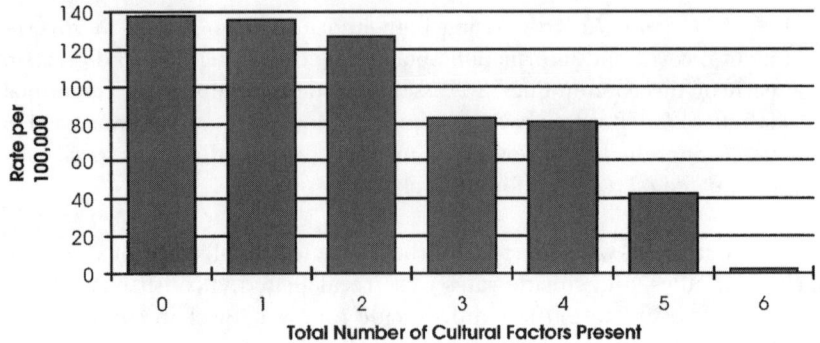

FIGURE 6.—Native youth suicide rates by number of factors present in the community (1987–1992).

community. When suicide rates were calculated for each score, the range extended from a high of 137.5 for the group of communities in which none of the markers were found to a low of zero for communities containing all six markers (see Figure 6). The staircase pattern evident in this figure was borne out statistically in a strong linear relation between suicide risk and the number of factors present ($\chi^2[6] = 10.042$, $p < 0.002$, Cramér's $V = 0.075$).

The point we take from these analyses is just this: The cases of youth suicides we observed were not randomly distributed across the nearly 200 separate communities that make up the First Nations population. Rather, variability in youth suicide rates can be better understood when viewed in light of the efforts these communities had made to preserve and promote their Native culture and to regain control over key aspects of their communal lives. If any doubt about this conclusion remained, the results from our recently completed second wave of data collection, this time covering the years 1993–2000, exhibited precisely this same stepwise function: Rates for communities with none of these markers far exceeded the provincial average; communities in which all markers were present continued to enjoy a complete absence of youth suicide (see Figure 7).

CONCLUSIONS

Our motivation for carrying out these epidemiological studies was to demonstrate that the concept of continuity may count as one of those rare social science concepts that proves useful at more than one level of analysis. Just as continuity at a *personal* level can provide a backstop to those moments when life might otherwise seem not worth living, and promotes the care and concern that we feel for our own individual futures, *cultural* continuity

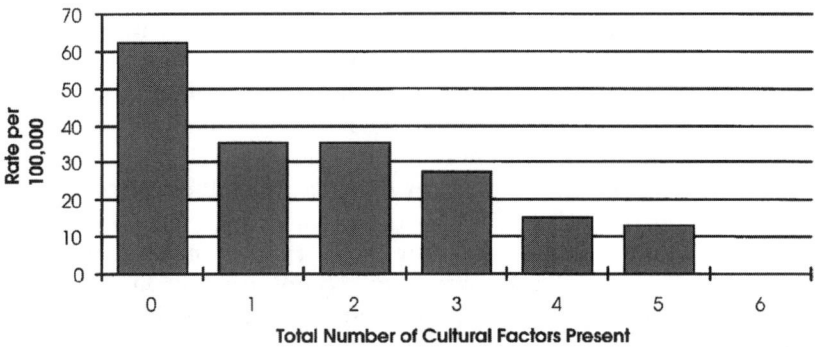

FIGURE 7.—Native youth suicide rates by number of factors present in the community (1993–2000).

represents a counterpart barometer of communal care and concern for a shared past and a collective future. Such care is reflected in efforts to preserve and promote cultural practices and to control and manage available resources in ways that conserve cultural identity in the face of acculturative forces. To the extent that all that is true—that efforts to "carry that ideal or conceptual future back into the present to create the sociocultural environment of the newcomer" (Cole, 1999, p. 88) really do form a cornerstone of psychological continuity—then community level efforts to promote cultural continuity ought to be reflected in the ability of young people to weather the storms of their own identity formation processes. Our data support this view: High scoring communities have low to vanishing youth suicide rates.

Of course, we don't mean to scare up ghosts from an intellectual past by suggesting that cultures can be rank ordered from least to most continuous in the same way it was once believed they could be classified from less to more developed (Tylor, 1874). We cannot resist the temptation, however, to note that Boas (1911), whose seminal work put the lie to this notion of cultural evolution, actually collected data from the same Rural Native community in which we gathered the self-continuity data reported in chapter VI. What distinguishes communities with little control over education is, for example, not a lack of will or want of effort. Current resources and barriers to progress vary widely across these communities. In much the same way, the historical harms visited upon Native people were not experienced by every First Nation in equal measure. Understanding the relation between measures of cultural continuity and indexes of individual continuity will obviously involve more than measuring these six marker variables and counting only the most tragic of failures in personal permanence. To that end, we are currently broadening our inquiry in two ways. First, under the guidance of First Nations community members, we are developing a set of more locally relevant measures of cultural continuity that catalog the particular responses of communities to their own unique conditions. Second, we are examining the impact of community efforts on the young people they are meant to protect and foster. Here we mean not only to gather reports from young persons concerning their perception of, or participation in, such efforts, but also to collect data on outcome measures other than suicide that (to our minds) ought to similarly reflect the protective value of cultural continuity: school completion rates and academic achievement on the upside, and injury and accident rates on the downside. All indications are that both new avenues of research will prove to be productive.

VI. CULTURE AS A SET POINT IN THE CHOICE BETWEEN NARRATIVIST AND ESSENTIALIST SELF-CONTINUITY WARRANTING PRACTICES

Chapter V concerned whole Aboriginal communities and the ways in which their shared efforts to collectively navigate matters of cultural continuity were related to the frequency of suicides among their own youth, just as chapter IV was also, in its own way, singular in its issues of identity and suicide in a different, although equally homogeneous, sample of culturally mainstream adolescents. When chapter III, which was no less about a largely seamless sample of rank-and-file public school children, is also thrown into the mix, it threatens to appear as though our version of cross-cultural research risks turning into the procedural equivalent of serial monogamy, oddly devoted to picking off different populations one culture at a time. The present chapter is not like that, and instead represents our best attempt at a direct comparison of the self-continuity warranting practices of various Aboriginal and non-Aboriginal samples.

STUDY FIVE: PERSONAL PERSISTENCE IN THE LIVES OF ABORIGINAL AND NON-ABORIGINAL YOUTH

This study differed in important ways from those described in the preceding chapters. First, although this study did not involve whole populations, as did chapter V, it was larger than the usual direct assessment studies. It involved lengthy, one-on-one interviews with more than 200 Native and non-Native youth drawn from three distinct communities, communities that differed one from the other in being more or less urban, or remote. It was also distinct from our other studies in that, unlike chapters III–V, which summarize findings that, though reanalyzed or otherwise augmented with new data, have already been detailed elsewhere, this study reports long strings of results, the particulars of which have so far been unpublished.

A third distinctive feature of the present study involves scoring. Although in chapter III we worked to frame and elaborate a distinction between Essentialist and Narrative approaches to the paradox of sameness and change, and gave equal pride of place to both of these distinctive problem-solving strategies, two chapters and three studies have now gone by with almost no mention of Narrative approaches to the dilemma of personal persistence. Responsibility for the lopsided emphasis on Essentialist solution strategies does not rest on any conviction of our own that such entity-based accounts are somehow inherently better or more adequate to the task of warranting continuity claims but rather on the cultural complexion of the Euro-American youth who participated in our initial studies. At least this was our orienting hypothesis at the beginning of the new work to be reported here, and, to anticipate our results, it is essentially the conclusion to which our cross-cultural research has led. That is, in chapters I and II we went to some lengths to argue the case that Western European culture, the culture from which the large bulk of the young persons who served as respondents in Studies One through Three were drawn, is committed first and foremost to an Essentialist view devoted to unearthing enduring and more genotypic parts lurking behind the phenotypic surface structures of what are taken to be largely ephemeral change. Things, or at least things of a natural kind, we are led to assume, almost always harbor some more or less abiding or more or less abstract or interiorized core of essential sameness (a hidden name or personality structure or immortal soul) that survives the ravages of time and can be pointed to when change threatens to cost us our continuity. To the degree that there is an element of truth in such common stereotypes, it need come as no great surprise that we could interview three studies worth of culturally mainstream adolescents without encountering a substantial number of young persons who could not be made to fit comfortably within that particular half of our scoring typology orchestrated to capture more or less sophisticated ways of being Essentialistic. In short, by capitalizing on samples of convenience drawn predominantly from the cultural mainstream we looked for and found a predominance of Essentialist thinking at every turn.

Notwithstanding the fact that such a situational explanation will largely do, some of the responsibility for having gotten this far with so little having yet been said about Narrative solutions to the problem of personal persistence is also owed to the fact that, having spent so much time looking where the light was brightest, we as a research team were no doubt initially slow to recognize instances of more Narrative approaches to the problem of personal persistence when they did occasionally arise. This is in part the reason, as we earlier attempted to make clear, that the more balanced descriptive typology (i.e., two tracks, Narrative and Essentialist—each with five levels) was the scoring scheme to which we eventually came, rather than the one with which we began. Eventually, with the benefit of hindsight and with the advantage of access to samples of young persons removed from the center of the cultural mainstream, the opportunity to observe and record the broad range of alternative solutions to the problem of personal persistence presented itself.

Belatedly armed with the emerging set of conceptual distinctions reflected in the scoring criteria elaborated in chapter II, gifted with the opportunity to interview substantial numbers of young persons reasonably representative of both Aboriginal and non-Aboriginal cultures, and informed by our earlier results based on interviews with rank-and-file adolescents of Euro-American descent, we approached the cross-cultural study now on report with the following set of hypotheses. First, because we had already found it to be true in the past, we anticipated that any new set of culturally mainstream adolescents would once again fall back onto what Polkinghorne (1988) called a "metaphysics of substance" and respond to questions about their own and others' personal persistence by adopting, as a default strategy, an Essentialist solution that followed one of the five levels detailed in our scoring typology. Our expectations for First Nations youth, on the other hand, were very different. Although Essentialist talk of "spirits" and more can certainly be heard in Native cultures, contemporary anthropologists (for a recent review of this literature see Bierwert, 1999) maintain that such references to essences commonly rest on a different metaphysical structure, one that does not regard such "spirits" as inhering to individuals (as does the Christian notion of a soul), but, instead, accords them a largely independent and autonomous existence (Bierwert, p. 176). In contrast, then, to any metaphysics of substances or essences often argued to dominate Western, Euro-American intellectual traditions, Native culture is broadly understood to adopt more of a metaphysics of "potentiality and actuality" (Polkinghorne; see also Deloria, 1979) that privileges becoming over being. All of this led us to hypothesize that First Nations youth, in contrast to their non-Native counterparts, would favor variations on what we have termed Narrative solutions to the problem of personal persistence.

Method

Participants

A total of 220 young persons participated. Respondents were drawn from three different communities: Rural Native ($N = 92$), Urban Native

($N = 91$), and non-Native ($N = 37$). Details of the numbers in each group appear below.

Rural Native sample. Participants from a Rural Native community, an island community located 30 miles off Canada's west coast, participated in two waves of data collection held 18 to 24 months apart. At Time 1, a total of 55 young persons were tested (32 females, 23 males; mean age = 15.25 years, age range = 12–20 years). All participants completed the Personal Persistence Interview which always began with one or more stories about persistence in the lives of others and always ended with an interview segment on self-continuity. Interview materials were presented in either print or film format. Those in the print condition ($N = 29$) read and heard a tape recorded version of a Native story (*Bear Woman*) and a non-Native story (*Valjean*). Those in the film condition ($N = 26$) watched a Native film (*Frank's Journey*) and a non-Native film (*Scrooge*). (These story materials are described in detail in the Materials and Procedures section below.) At Time 2, a total of 67 young persons were tested (35 females, 32 males, range = 12–22 years mean age = 16.78 years). Forty-two of these young persons completed the Personal Persistence Interview. For reasons detailed in the Results section, the story materials used with this follow-up group were presented in print format only, with one Native story (*Bear Woman*) and one non-Native story (*Valjean*). These 42 participants, along with an additional sample of 25 available volunteers, also completed a four-part Questionnaire Battery (described in the Materials and Procedures section).

Urban Native sample. This sample was composed of members of a band whose traditional lands are located on the apron of a major west coast Canadian city. A total of 91 young persons from this community (51 females, 40 males; mean age = 15.31 years, age range = 13–18 years) either completed the Personal Persistence Interview ($N = 65$) or the Questionnaire Battery ($N = 26$) or both ($N = 2$). Those who completed the Personal Persistence Interview received stories in either print ($N = 32$, *Bear Woman, Valjean*) or film format ($N = 35$; *Frank's Journey, Scrooge*).

Non-Native sample. Beyond choosing young persons of similar ages, there was no obvious collection of non-Native youth that constituted an ideal study group against which to compare the responses of our Native samples. Direct socioeconomic comparisons between persons who do and do not live on federal reserves are naturally suspect, as would be any attempt to draw parallels with other minority groups. The closest thing to a theory-relevant prospect was judged to be a sample of adolescents whose cultural roots run as deep as possible into traditional

Euro-American culture, a possibility not easily realized in the multicultural context of an urban, Pacific rim city. The sample eventually settled on was one drawn from a suburban, lower middle class parochial school maintained by the descendents of what, a century ago, was a Dutch Reform immigrant group. A total of 37 youth (18 females, 19 males; mean age = 15.73 years, range = 13–18 years) were recruited from this school and completed the Personal Persistence Interview using story materials in either print ($N = 18$, *Bear Woman*, *Valjean*) or film ($N = 19$, *Frank's Journey*, *Scrooge*) format.

Materials and Procedures

All interviews were conducted in the participants' home communities. Questionnaire data, where obtained, were collected during the same session in which interviews were held. Within the Native communities, permission to enter traditional territories and to make use of community facilities was obtained from the Chief and Band council. For the non-Native sample, permission was obtained from the school principal and from classroom teachers.

Personal Persistence Interview. As described in chapter III, the Personal Persistence Interview was designed to gather participants' thoughts concerning continuity in their own life (the Self portion) and in the lives of the protagonists in Native and non-Native films and stories. Four stories were used: two drawn from Western literary tradition (Victor Hugo's *Les Misérables*, and Charles Dickens' *A Christmas Carol*) and two were selected for their Native content (*The Girl Who Lived with the Bears*, a traditional Haida story published in the form of a children's book by Diamond Goldin & Plewes in 1997, and *Jan Ah Dah—It Hurts*, a film produced by Northern Native Broadcasting, a First Nations company in the Yukon Territory, concerning a Native adolescent's struggle following the death of a friend). These stories were then rendered into either picture book or video format for presentation to our young participants. The print stories were modeled on *Classic Comic Books*: minimal text accompanied by color illustrations. A Classic Comics version of *Les Misérables* was adapted for use in the procedure by eliminating certain sections of the story to produce a 24-page color booklet we referred to as *Valjean*. The Native story, *The Girl Who Lived with the Bears*, was similarly shortened and referred to as *Bear Woman*. The text of each comic was then recorded on audio cassette and played aloud as the participant read the story. These recordings were approximately 10 minutes in length. The 1951 film version of *A Christmas Carol* (*Scrooge*, starring Alastair Sim) was edited to produce a 10-minute video tape. The Native film *Jan Ah Dah*

—*It Hurts* was similarly edited to produce a 10-minute video tape we referred to as *Frank's Journey*.

Participants read/heard (or watched) the story and were then asked to provide descriptions of the main character as she or he appeared at the beginning and then at the end of the story (see the Appendix for the standardized text and probe questions used in these interviews). The thrust of the interview protocol was to draw attention to the differences in these earlier and later portions of these accounts, and to urge the participant to explain why or how it was that these two very different descriptions could apply to the same person (e.g., "What was Valjean like at the beginning of the story?" "What was Monsieur Madeleine like at the end of the story?" "Why, despite the very different ways that you describe them, do you believe that Valjean and Monsieur Madeleine are one and the same person?"). Where necessary, standard probe questions were used to urge the participants to expand on their explanations. Thoughts concerning continuity in the participants' own life were obtained in similar fashion by asking the young persons to describe themselves at some point in the past (5 to10 years earlier, depending on their current age) and then asking for a current self-description (see the Appendix). Differences in these descriptions were then underscored and the participant was asked how these could apply to the same person. Again, standardized probe questions were used if the explanations were judged to be too brief. Individual interviews were completed in a single 60–90 minute session and recorded on audio tape for later transcription.

Questionnaire battery. Our four-part paper-and-pencil questionnaire battery was constructed using items from several existing measures. Part 1 of the battery was Kuhn and McPartland's (1954) *Twenty Statements Test* (TST) also known as the "Who am I?" test. The TST consists of 20 sentence stems, all beginning with the phrase: "I am...." Participants are asked to complete the phrases in whatever ways they deem fit. Part 2 was Singelis' (1994) *Self-Construal Scale*, a 24-item questionnaire for assessing individuals' Independent and Interdependent self-construals. Part 3 was Dweck's (2000) *Implicit Theories of Personality Scale*, a set of six statements concerning personality and personality change that respondent's rate according to a five-step agree-disagree scale. Part 4 was a 130-item Ethnic Identification Scale constructed from four other measures: (a) the *Vancouver Index of Acculturation* (VIA; Ryder, Alden, & Paulhus, 2000), a self-report instrument that assesses several domains relevant to acculturation, including values, social relationships, and adherence to traditions; (b) Ward and Rana-Deuba's (1999) *Acculturation Index*, which assesses two dimensions (host and conational identification) and four modes (integration, separation, marginalization, and assimilation) of acculturation; (c) Phinney's (1992) *Multigroup Ethnic Identity Measure* (MEIM), a questionnaire measure designed for use across diverse ethnic groups; and, (d) Zygmuntowiscz et al.'s (2000) *Values Orientation Scale*, a version of an earlier measure by Szapocznik, Scopetta, Kurtines, and Aranalde (1978) that has been specifically adapted for use with Canadian Aboriginal youth. Questionnaires were completed either immediately preceding or following the Personal Persistence Interview (for those who attended an interview) or during a single session for those who were not interviewed.

Results

Before searching out possible differences in the performance of our Native and non-Native groups, we first needed to be convinced that our assessment procedures were comfortably within the competence range of our participants, and that none of the various experimental conditions or testing materials we had employed worked to especially handicap any relevant subset of the young persons tested. For that reason, we begin by reporting the results from a series of background statistical analyses meant to shore up our trust that the data were appropriate for answering the larger questions for which our studies were designed. First, we searched for potential differences in the ages and gender distributions of the various subgroups of participants, and then we examined participant attrition and response rates as indexes of task difficulty. This was followed by analyses of the variance that arose from the use of different story materials and display media employed in different iterations of our interview procedure. Having satisfied ourselves that the data could be relied on to pass these necessary quality assurance tests, we turned, in the analyses that followed, to issues of interrater reliability in the scoring of the interview transcripts, all before coming to the real heart of the matter: comparing the types of reasoning used by our research participants, and the various factors that might influence those judgments.

Demographic Characteristics of the Sample: Age and Gender

A total of 179 young persons (81 male, 98 female) completed the Personal Persistence Interview (either at Time 1 [$N = 160$], Time 2 [$N = 42$], or both [$N = 23$]). Of these, 142 were First Nations (77 Rural Native, 65 Urban Native) and 37 were non-Native. The mean ages of these groups at the time of their first interview are shown in Table 5. No reliable age differences were intended or found across the groups, nor between the genders with the exception that within the Rural Native group the female

TABLE 5

PARTICIPANT MEAN AGE (AND STANDARD DEVIATIONS) BY GROUP AND GENDER

Group	Overall		Male		Female	
	N	Age	N	Age	N	Age
Native	142	15.30 (2.16)	62	15.21 (2.13)	80	15.37 (2.20)
Rural Native	77	15.26 (2.47)	34	14.76 (2.37)	43	15.65 (2.51)
Urban Native	65	15.35 (1.74)	28	15.75 (1.67)	37	15.75 (1.67)
Non-Native	37	15.73 (1.50)	19	16.11 (1.66)	18	15.33 (1.24)
Total	179	15.39 (2.05)	81	15.42 (2.05)	98	15.37 (2.05)

TABLE 6

RATIO OF MALE TO FEMALE PARTICIPANTS BY GROUP

Group	Male : Female
Native	.77:1
Rural Native	.79:1
Urban Native	.76:1
Non-Native	1.05:1
Total	.83:1

participants who took part in the follow-up interview (Time 2) were reliably older than their male counterparts ($F = 17.1$ years; $M = 15.2$ years; $F(1, 49) = 6.254$ $p = .02$), a fact due, in all likelihood, to the tendency for older First Nation males to leave reserve communities in search of employment.

Although slightly more females than males were interviewed, the distribution of gender across groups did not otherwise deviate from what would be expected by chance (see Table 6). This held true across the three communities ($\chi^2_{[2]} = .985$, $p = .611$), as well as for the combined Native versus non-Native groups ($\chi^2_{[1]} = .701, p = .460$).

Indexes of Task Difficulty: Subject Attrition and Data Integrity

Our assessment procedures included materials drawn from two cultural sources (Native and non-Native) and presented in two formats (print and video). Given the differences in the cultural backgrounds of our participants, we were concerned that some of the young people might find some of the materials more interesting or more difficult than others, perhaps in systematic ways that could work to bias our findings.

Consequently, we needed assurances that the procedures were not too "foreign" or technically demanding, or otherwise inappropriate in ways that might differentially affect performance or participant attrition within our cultural groups, causing those who survived to be unrepresentative of the age or cultural groups from which they were drawn. A set of analyses was conducted to inspect these possibilities, beginning with an examination of those relatively rare cases in which our interview data proved unusable.

A total of 202 interview transcripts were scored (23 participants interviewed at both Time 1 and Time 2, 137 interviewed only at T1, and 19 only at T2). Each participant's transcript contained data derived from the discussion of either two or three stimulus stories. Of the resulting total pool of 554 story transcripts, 41 (7.4%) were judged to contain too little data to be reliably coded and so were classified as "unscorable." For the most part, these stories (not participants) were excluded because of recording equipment failure or because the interview was interrupted or otherwise incomplete. In several cases, however, two raters concluded that, despite our best efforts, the young persons involved had provided too little information in response to questioning on that particular story to allow a confident rating of their reasoning.

Of the 41 story transcripts judged unscorable, 13 were provided by just five participants whose complete interview protocols contained no scorable data whatsoever. With these 5 participants removed from the data set, the rates of unscorable stories were 3 of 110 (2.7%) stories from our non-Native participants and 25 of 431 (5.8%) from Native participants. As such, no remarkable or statistically significant difference was observed between groups in terms of the frequency of unscorable stories ($\chi^2_{[1]} = 1.69, p = .19$), nor were any sex differences found (males = 15 of 249, females = 13 of 289; $\chi^2_{[1]} = 1.06, p = .30$).

Content and Media Effects

Our scoring procedures were designed to produce a Track (I or II) and Level (1–5) classification for each story. Because later analyses centered on overall summary scores derived for each participant across stories that differed in content (Native, non-Native, Self) and presentation media (book, video), it was important to rule out the possibility that subsequent classifications might have been differentially influenced by these factors.

Story content. There is some question about the wisdom of comparing Level across Tracks. That is, because these are categorical rather than continuous data, it is not clear that the designation "Level 2" carries the same meaning on both Track I and Track II. Nevertheless,

TABLE 7

MEAN PERSONAL PERSISTENCE LEVEL SCORES BY STORY TYPE

Story Type	Mean Level Score (SD)
Native	2.665 (1.161)
Non-native	2.719 (1.195)
Self	2.622 (1.127)

Note.—$N = 127$.

TABLE 8

MEAN PERSONAL PERSISTENCE LEVEL SCORES BY STORY TYPE AND TRACK

Story Type	Essentialist Track (SD)	Narrative Track (SD)
Native	2.547 (1.395)	2.691 (1.518)
Non-native	2.726 (1.449)	2.845 (1.658)
Self	2.597 (1.244)	2.600 (1.588)

Note.—$N = 89$.

simply assuming a rough equivalence by treating these data points as though they constitute an ordinal scale (regardless of track), a total of 127 participants produced scorable data on all three story types (Native, non-Native, Self). These were collapsed across Tracks, and the mean Level scores assigned appear in Table 7. No significant differences were found across story types in terms of the Level classifications ($F(2, 250) = 0.435$, ns).

An analysis that compared the Level scores separately for each Track across story types for those participants who were consistently given the same Track assignment ($N = 89$) was also undertaken. Again, there were no significant differences in mean Level scores based on the content of the stories: ($F(2, 54) = 0.400$, $p = 0.672$ for Essentialists, $F(2, 116) = 0.690$, $p = 0.504$ for Narrativists; see Table 8).

In testing these Group by Story differences, the between-group factor Native versus non-Native was included to search for possible interactions between the cultural content of the story and the cultural background of the participants. None of these interactions were found to be statistically significant.

What these analyses tell us is that our participants' Level scores were not, as we were cautiously concerned they might be, substantially influenced by the particular content of the stories, nor by the extent to which that content could be considered "consistent" with the participants' cultural background. Consequently, it was judged appropriate to collapse across such story content differences in subsequent analyses.

TABLE 9

MEAN PERSONAL PERSISTENCE LEVEL SCORES (AND STANDARD DEVIATIONS) BY STORY CONTENT AND PRESENTATION MEDIUM

Story Content	Presentation Medium	
	Video	Comic
Native	2.526 (1.147)	2.366 (1.146)
Non-Native	2.421 (1.184)	2.537 (1.178)

Note.—$N = 79$.

Media effects. A series of analyses was then conducted in an effort to test whether any individual story or presentation medium (print vs. video) was differentially related to participants' responses. To compare the possible effects of presentational media, a 2×2 (Between Groups × Within Stories) ANOVA was computed using only the data from the non-Native and Rural Native participants tested at Time 1. The analysis was limited to data from those participants for whom media constituted a between factor in the design (individual participants received all stories in the same media, either video or comic), and story content was a within factor (all subjects received one Native and one non-Native story, with the order counterbalanced). The mean Level scores by content and media type are shown in Table 9. Despite our initial concern that some of our participant groups might be adversely affected by the challenges of print media, no such effect for media was found: $F_{(1,77)} = .008$, $p = .927$; nor was there a difference by story content (Native, non-Native, $F(1, 77) = .122, p = .728$), nor any interaction among these factors: $F(1, 77) = 2.167, p = .145$. Because no differences based on media or content were found in this large subset of our data, subsequent interviews conducted with urban Native participants and interviews at Time 2 were not blocked on this factor.

A comparison across all participants similarly showed that scores did not differ on the Native video versus the Native comic (mean scores were 2.606 and 2.348, respectively): $t(158) = -1.563, p = .12$; nor did scores differ for the non-Native video and non-Native comic (mean scores 2.610 and 2.438, respectively): Welch's $t(139.48) = .994, p = .32$. Finally, no sex differences were found in scores examined by media or story content.

Interrater Reliability

Our procedures involved the testing of 179 young people. As described above, 5 were excluded from analysis due to concerns about the quality of

TABLE 10
INTERRATER AGREEMENT WITH RESPECT TO PERSONAL PERSISTENCE TRACK ASSIGNMENT

Story Type	Agreement Rate	Kappa
Native	96 of 112 (85.7%)	.673*
Non-Native	85 of 103 (82.5%)	.631*
Self	98 of 114 (85.6%)	.714*
Total	279 of 329 (84.8%)	.675*

Note.—*$p < .0005$.

TABLE 11
CROSS-RATER CLASSIFICATION OF PERSONAL PERSISTENCE TRACK ASSIGNMENTS

		Rater 1			
		Essentialist	Narrative	Unscorable	Total
Rater 2	Essentialist	70	29	0	99
	Narrative	9	199	3	211
	Unscorable	4	5	10	19
	Total	83	233	13	329

the data, and 23 were interviewed at both Time 1 and Time 2. In total, then (counting those who were tested on more than one occasion), we obtained 197 interview transcripts containing 541 separate stories. To assess interrater reliability, a subset of 115 of the 197 transcripts (58.4%) chosen at random were scored independently by two raters. These transcripts contained a total of 329 stories. Each story was twice classified according to track (Track I = Essentialist, Track II = Narrative), and within each track the stories were assigned one of five levels. The analyses reported below were meant to determine how often our raters assigned the same Track or Level classification across the assessment opportunities that were afforded (2 or 3 stimulus stories, and 1 or 2 testing sessions). Rates of interrater agreement are reported separately for Track and Level assignments.

Agreement on Track ratings. Our raters agreed in their assessment of Track in 285 of the 335 stories (84.8%, Cohen's kappa = .68, $p < .0005$). Rates of agreement were uniformly high across the three types of stories (see Table 10). Table 11 displays these same ratings cross-tabulated, with cases of agreement appearing on the diagonal.

Agreement on Level ratings. As noted above, it makes questionable sense to count as cases of interrater agreement those instances in which

TABLE 12

INTERRATER AGREEMENT WITH RESPECT TO PERSONAL PERSISTENCE LEVEL ASSIGNMENTS

Level Assignment	Number of cases	(%)
Agreed	239	(85.6)
Disagreed by 1 level	31	(11.1)
Disagreed by 2 levels	7	(2.5)
Disagreed by 3 levels	2	(0.7)
Disagreed by 4 levels	0	(0)

TABLE 13

INTERRATER AGREEMENT WITH RESPECT TO PERSONAL PERSISTENCE LEVEL ASSIGNMENTS BY STORY TYPE

Story Type	Agreement Rate	Kappa
Native	83 of 96 (86.5%)	.778*
Non-Native	70 of 85 (82.4%)	.750*
Self	86 of 98 (87.6%)	.820*
Total	239 of 279 (85.7%)	.786*

Note.—*$p < .0005$.

participants were given the same Level but different Track assignments. Therefore, attention was restricted to that subset of 279 stories where the two raters agreed in their Track classifications. Of these, raters agreed in their Level classification on 239 of 279 stories that they jointly considered (85.7%, Cohen's kappa = .786, $p < .0005$). The extent of disagreement was also minimal: In 96.8% of all cases, the raters either agreed or were within one Level of agreement (see Table 12). Table 13 shows the interrater agreement by Story Type.

Within-Subject Consistency and Summary Ratings

Our interpretative framework did not require that participants be consistent across occasions. Rather, we assumed that all of our participants were in fact capable of responding in either an Essentialist or Narrative fashion, or otherwise had "access" to these two distinct ways of proceeding, but that for various reasons, including possible cultural reasons of the sort featured in this *Monograph*, they ordinarily employed one or the other of these continuity-preserving warranting strategies as a default option. As such, it was our strong expectation that, although not obligated to do so, most participants would ordinarily respond in ways coded as being

TABLE 14

Participant Consistency with Respect to Personal Persistence Level Assignments
(1–5)

Level Assignment	Number of Cases (%)
Consistent	115 (58.4)
Varied by 1 level	46 (23.3)
Varied by 2 levels	32 (16.2)
Varied by 3 levels	4 (2.0)
Varied by 4 levels	0 (0)

representative of the same Track across the several story problems they undertook. If this were not so—that is, if responding in either a Narrative or Essentialist fashion on one occasion had no bearing on the likelihood of being coded in a similar fashion on subsequent occasions—then there would be no point in going on to speculate about how culture or anything else might systematically influence Track assignment. Consequently, it was judged important to determine whether the participants in the present study sequence would respond in the same or different ways when required to respond to interview questions about discontinuities in their own life and the lives of other Native and non-Native story characters. This same analysis acquired additional importance because of our initial intention and eventual practice of deriving a single Track and Level classification for each participant: a global classification that summed across these various data sources and that presupposed a reasonable degree of consistency of the sort just described. The "within-subject consistency" analyses reported below worked to help justify this summary rating.

A total of 149 of 197 (75.6%) participants were found to be totally consistent in their Track assignments across all stories. In other words, 3 out of 4 participants displayed the same Track on all of the stories (mean of 2.75 stories per participant, standard deviation of 0.50). The remaining 48 participants were assigned the Track associated with their most sophisticated level of reasoning. Clearly, although "access" to both sorts of warranting strategies was frequently demonstrated, most participants did have a default strategy that was regularly exercised.

For Level of reasoning, about which our theoretical expectations were less strong, 115 of 197 participants (58.4%) consistently used the same Track and Level of reasoning across all of the stories. For the remaining 82 participants, their highest Level was used for the overall rating. Table 14 displays the degree to which participants were consistent in their reasoning. Obviously, more often than not, a participant's use of a given response strategy scored at a given coding Level was the best available predictor of how he or she would respond on subsequent occasions.

TABLE 15

PERSONAL PERSISTENCE TRACK ASSIGNMENTS BY GENDER, GROUP, AND COMMUNITY

	Essentialist	Narrative
Gender		
Male	25 (31.6%)	54 (68.3%)
Female	22 (23.2%)	73 (76.8%)
Group		
Native	19 (13.9%)	118 (86.1%)
Non-Native	28 (75.7%)	9 (24.3%)
Community		
Rural Native	10 (13.9%)	62 (86.1%)
Urban Native	9 (13.8%)	56 (86.2%)
Non-Native	28 (75.7%)	9 (24.3%)

Taken together, these analyses went some important distance in assuring us that the responses of our participants could be consistently located within our two-track, five-level coding scheme.

Factors Associated With Track and Level Assignments

As described above, for each interview the participants were given a Track and Level assignment for each of the stories presented and a Track and Level assignment for the discussion of continuity in their own life. In the following subsections we report on a series of analyses that searched for factors associated with these assignments. These analyses focused on four factors (age, gender, cultural group, and community) and are reported separately for Track and Level classifications.

Track. As anticipated on theoretical grounds, the groups did differ dramatically in that Native participants were much more likely to be classified as Track II (Narrative) and non-Native participants were particularly likely to be classified as Track I (Essentialist): $\chi^2_{[1]} = 56.448$, $p < .005$, Cramér's $V = 0.570$ (see Table 15). The Native communities themselves did not, however, differ from one another in the frequency of Narrative or Essentialist ratings ($\chi^2_{[1]} = 0$, $p < .994$). Track assignments were not associated with age differences: $F[1, 172] = .495, p = .483$. (Track 1: 15.6; Track 2: 15.4) nor with gender ($\chi^2_{[1]} = 1.576, p < .209$).

Level. Two methods of calculating an overall Level score were used: an Average Level score (the mean of Level scores across stories that were assigned the same Track) and a Highest Level score.

TABLE 16
HIGHEST MEAN PERSONAL PERSISTENCE LEVEL SCORES (AND STANDARD DEVIATIONS) BY TRACK AND GENDER

Group	Essentialist	Narrative	Total
Male	2.840 (1.344)	2.444 (0.904)	2.570 (1.070)
Female	3.318 (1.359)	2.836 (0.727)	2.947 (0.926)
Native	2.579 (1.305)	2.661 (0.808)	2.650 (0.888)
Non-Native	3.393 (1.315)	2.778 (1.093)	3.243 (1.278)
Total	3.063 (1.358)	2.669 (0.827)	2.776 (1.009)

Because of the unequal numbers of participants within our groups, separate analyses of each respondent's Highest Level score were conducted for the Narrative and Essentialist groups. Each of these analyses examined the relation of cultural background (Native vs. non-Native) and gender to Level scores. In each analysis, participants were randomly removed from the data set to achieve proportionality across the groups. With age partialled out, reliable differences emerged only within the Narrative group. On average, non-Native Narrativists had higher Level ratings than Native Narrativists (adjusted means: 3.204 vs. 2.634) and Female Narrativists had higher Level ratings than Male Narrativists (adjusted means: 3.103 vs. 2.735). No differences were found within the Essentialist group. In subsequent analyses, special care was taken to control for these ancillary effects.

To determine whether differences existed *between* the Narrative and Essentialist groups, a final ANCOVA was computed in which gender, age, and cultural group were partialled out. No reliable differences in highest level score were observed between the Narrative and Essentialists.

Analyzing the data by community, a reliable difference for level scores emerged: The Rural Native community had lower scores than the Urban Native and Urban non-Native groups, who did not differ from one another ($F[2, 171] = 11.304$, $p < .0005$, partial $\eta^2 = 0.117$, Tukey's HSD; see Tables 16 and 17).

When overall Level was calculated by averaging individual Level scores within the participants' overall Track assignment, no reliable differences were observed by gender or group and no reliable interaction was observed between these factors (see Table 18). Again, a reliable difference by community emerged, with the Rural Native community scoring lower than the others ($F[2, 171] = 7.199$, $p < .001$, partial $\eta^2 = 0.078$, Tukey's HSD; see Table 19).

Significant positive correlations between age and Level score were (as expected) observed for both highest Level ($r = .32$, $p < .0005$, $r^2 = .10$) and average Level ($r = .27$, $p < .0005$, $r^2 = .07$).

TABLE 17
HIGHEST MEAN PERSONAL PERSISTENCE LEVEL SCORES (AND STANDARD DEVIATIONS) BY COMMUNITY

Group	Rural Native	Urban Native	Non-Native	Total
Male	2.000 (1.016)	2.821 (0.670)	3.158 (1.214)	2.570 (1.070)
Female	2.700 (0.853)	3.027 (0.645)	3.333 (1.372)	2.947 (0.926)
Essentialist	2.300 (1.142)	2.889 (1.167)	3.393 (1.315)	3.063 (1.358)
Narrative	2.403 (0.913)	2.946 (0.553)	2.778 (1.093)	2.669 (0.827)
Total	2.389 (0.987)	2.939 (0.659)	3.243 (1.278)	2.776 (1.009)

TABLE 18
MEAN PERSONAL PERSISTENCE LEVEL SCORES (AND STANDARD DEVIATIONS) BY TRACK AND GROUP

Group	Essentialist	Narrative	Total
Male	2.467 (1.175)	2.244 (0.855)	2.314 (0.965)
Female	2.902 (1.220)	2.573 (0.664)	2.649 (0.831)
Native	2.421 (1.267)	2.421 (0.754)	2.421 (0.837)
Non-Native	2.839 (1.151)	2.593 (0.943)	2.779 (1.096)
Total	2.670 (1.203)	2.433 (0.766)	2.497 (0.907)

TABLE 19
MEAN PERSONAL PERSISTENCE LEVEL SCORES (AND STANDARD DEVIATIONS) BY COMMUNITY

Group	Rural Native	Urban Native	Non-Native	Total
Male	1.885 (0.938)	2.530 (0.722)	2.719 (1.080)	2.314 (0.965)
Female	2.454 (0.804)	2.766 (0.641)	2.843 (1.141)	2.649 (0.831)
Essentialist	2.100 (1.296)	2.778 (1.202)	2.839 (1.151)	2.670 (1.203)
Narrative	2.218 (0.840)	2.646 (0.573)	2.593 (0.943)	2.433 (0.766)
Total	2.201 (0.906)	2.664 (0.682)	2.779 (1.096)	2.497 (0.907)

Stability and Temporal Consistency of Reasoning (Longitudinal Data)

If, as hypothesized, culture is a primary determinant of whether one's default strategy in solving problems of personal persistence is principally Narrative or Essentialist, then, short of some cultural overhaul, a respondent's Track assignment ought not to be variable but generally enduring across substantial intervals of time. As a preliminary test of this hypothesis, a small longitudinal study was carried out. Eighteen to 24 months following our initial interviews, 23 of the young participants from the Rural Native community were located and reinterviewed. Because analysis of the data from Time 1 indicated no differences between groups according to presentation medium or story content, the testing materials at Time 2 were represented only in comic book format. Again, the stories contained both Native and non-Native characters and were followed by a discussion of continuity in the participant's own life. The analyses reported below concern the consistency of the participants' reasoning across this two-year time window.

Consistency With Respect to Track

The proportion of participants using Narrative reasoning in this all-Native sample increased from 67% at Time 1 to 87% at Time 2. At the time of the initial interview, 20 of 23 respondents consistently employed one type of reasoning (either Essentialist or Narrative) with reference to the personal persistence of the various story characters and in discussing their own lives. During the follow-up interview, 22 of 23 respondents were consistent in the type of reasoning used. Overall, 16 of 23 (70%) employed the same type of general self-continuity warranting strategy across both testing sessions.

Consistency With Respect to Level

Fourteen of 23 participants exhibited the same Level of reasoning throughout the first interview (i.e., across all the stories within that interview). Fifteen of 23 did so at the second interview. Across both testing sessions, just under half of these young persons (11 of 23) employed the same level of reasoning on each and every story during both interviews.

Changes in Reasoning Level from Time 1 to Time 2

If, as predicted, adolescents ordinarily become increasingly sophisticated in their solutions to the problem of sameness in the face of personal change, then at least some of those tested could be expected to shift the level of their explanations during the two-year interval covered by this study. Of the 16 respondents whose consistent use of the same type of continuity argument allowed such change scores to be calculated, exactly half showed this hypothesized pattern of improvement. Of the remaining 8 respondents, 2 showed a measurable but trivial decline and the remainder stayed the same. Those whose level did not change were either already at ceiling (Level 5) on the scale at Time 1 (four participants) or at floor (Level 1) at Time 1 (two of our youngest subjects) and were rated at Level 1 during both interviews. Even within this restricted sample of 16 participants, we observed a strong statistical trend toward increasingly higher scoring levels over time, $t(30) = 2.092$ (one-tailed), $p = .054$, Cohen's $\Delta = 0.424$.

Although these numbers are too small to warrant elaborate statistical analyses, it is obvious by inspection that, as anticipated, real change did take place for an important number of these young participants, and when it did it was most often in the direction of greater complexity.

Measures of Linguistic Sophistication

In the arguments presented above, we have endeavored to make a convincing case that there really are at least two fundamentally different strategies that young people (sometimes even the same people) utilize in coming to grips with the paradox of sameness and change, and this contention was strongly supported by our data. Young Native participants disproportionately employed Narrative self-continuity warranting strategies, and their non-Native counterparts most often displayed a default strategy that is Essentialist in character. Although it was our intention to lay this difference at the door of the different cultures of which these young people are a part, it remained possible that the findings were instead the coincidental byproduct of some more mundane set of factors. Because of such possibilities, it was necessary to strengthen our case by also exploring and, where possible, discounting other typically more reductive explanations for the pattern of our results. In other words, we wanted to rule out unnecessarily reductive readings of Narrative or Essentialist self-continuity arguments, or, more pointedly, we wanted, if possible, to rule out the prospect that the Narrative responses were simply Essentialist answers offered by those without a gift for abstraction, or that the Essentialist responses were simply Narrative answers put forward by those without a sense of plot.

We first examined the possibility that our coding of Narrativism versus Essentialism might not indicate deeply different ways of thinking about personal persistence, but rather might represent an artifact of something like different linguistic styles or abilities. Such an argument assumes (in contrast to our own claims) that one of these strategies is simply better than the other, and that our coding of these young people as either Narrativists or Essentialists was merely an indication of some more or less mature understanding of the self-continuity paradox. Given the predictable Euro-American bias in favor of Essentialist forms of reasoning, the canonical version of such a dismissive argument would be that Narrativity is simply a "problem" that will go away with sufficient Westernization. To put this argument to the test, the text of each of the transcripts of the Personal

TABLE 20

MEANS (AND STANDARD DEVIATIONS) OF MEASURES OF LINGUISTIC COMPLEXITY BY GROUP

Variable	Group	
	Essentialist	Narrative
Word count*	1204.05 (944.01)	829.79 (655.22)
Words per sentence	11.75 (5.40)	10.86 (6.04)
Words >6 letters	11.32 (2.01)	11.54 (2.22)
Cognitive process words	8.45 (2.22)	8.45 (2.36)
Causation words	1.29 (0.76)	1.48 (0.71)
Insight words	2.70 (0.95)	2.86 (1.38)
Discrepancy words	2.60 (1.05)	2.40 (1.16)
Inhibition words	0.14 (0.17)	0.15 (0.24)
Tentative words	3.73 (1.77)	3.84 (1.67)
Certainty words	1.11 (0.55)	0.99 (0.65)

Note.—*Significant Group difference, Cohen's $\Delta = 0.444$ ($\alpha = 0.02$).

Persistence Interview was stripped of interviewer comments and meticulously combed to properly mark and discard nonfluencies (e.g., "um") and fillers (e.g., "ya know") that might otherwise mislead our analysis. These sanitized transcripts were then analyzed using Pennebaker's *Linguistic Inquiry and Word Count* (LIWC) text analysis program. The LIWC analyzes a total of 74 predetermined linguistic variables for any given sample of text (Pennebaker & King, 1999). The LIWC was chosen because of its proven success with such analyses in general (Pennebaker & Graybeal, 2001) and because of its demonstrated utility in assessing cognitive and linguistic complexity (Pennebaker & Lay, 2002; Pennebaker & Stone, in press). This earlier research also served to guide our choice of 10 particular marker variables selected as a measure of cognitive and linguistic sophistication: word count, number of words per sentence, number of words longer than six letters, words related to cognitive processes (e.g., cause, know), causation words (e.g., because, effect), words commenting on insight (e.g., think, consider), words connoting a discrepancy (e.g., should, could), inhibition words (e.g., block, constrain), tentative words (e.g., maybe, perhaps), and certainty words (e.g., always, never).

All Western biases in favor of Essentialism notwithstanding, no remarkable differences were observed between the Narrativists and Essentialists on 9 of these 10 cognitive and linguistic complexity measures (Table 20). Perhaps ironically, our Essentialists were (on average) somewhat more wordy, but otherwise no more complex, than their Narrativist counterparts.

Although there is no simple way of knowing with numerical certainty, this result was likely due to cultural differences in the ways Native and non-

Native youth often express themselves. Our informal experience in interviewing more than 300 young people suggested that Native youth tended to be much more circumspect with their words, at least when being formally interviewed by adult representatives of a different culture, an impression that was given some support by our word-count data: $t'(38.835) = 2.733$, $p = 0.009$, Cohen's $\Delta = 0.524$. This finding should not, however, be taken to imply that the differences observed between those scored as Essentialists and as Narrativist (whatever their culture of origin) can be accounted for by simple verbal facility. When the same linguistic analyses were conducted separately for the two cultural groups, this difference disappeared, leaving no significant differences between Narrativists and Essentialists on any of the 10 marker variables of linguistic sophistication. Such a pattern of results strongly supported our contention that neither of these warranting strategies is merely a less sophisticated or inferior version of the other, and that they are equal in complexity and only different in application.

Having said this, it comes as no surprise that age was significantly related to many of these 10 marker variables in the Pennebaker measure because it is reasonable to expect that older participants would be more linguistically and cognitively complex than their younger counterparts. Likewise, it was not surprising that our better-advantaged non-Native sample did slightly better on some of these variables than did our Native sample. What is more interesting, however, is how these markers of linguistic ability related to our level-of-reasoning classifications. That is, we wish to preemptively counter what amounts to the opposite criticism that we just defended against concerning warranting strategy or type. More specifically, it could be reductively argued that what we saw as more or less sophisticated ways of justifying continuity within each Track actually amounted to no more than trivial linguistic styles that did not reflect real differences in the complexity of the arguments on offer. It seemed important, then, to establish whether or not (irrespective of Track) each successive level of reasoning represented a more sophisticated way of justifying self-continuity by examining the association between Level and other measures of cognitive and linguistic sophistication.

Because our level classifications were also highly correlated with age ($r = 0.361$, $p < 0.0005$, $r^2 = .130$), effects of age were partialled out of the relations we observed between the Pennebaker variables and our level classifications and, in view of the fact that there were 10 such correlations, we evaluated them at a reduced alpha level ($\alpha = 0.02$). In these analyses, 5 of the 10 variables showed significant correlations between level and complexity, and three additional variables demonstrated strong trends (see Table 21). Interestingly, when age was correlated with these 10 variables, and level was partialled out, "words per sentence" was the only variable also related

TABLE 21

Correlations Between Measures of Linguistic Complexity and Level and Age

Variable	Level (with Age partialled out)	Age (with Level partialled out)
Word count	$r = .49, p < .001, r^2 = .24$*	$r = .15, p < .055$
Words per sentence	$r = .30, p < .001, r^2 = .09$*	$r = .22, p < .005, r^2 = .05$*
Words >6 letters	$r = .14, p < .078$	$r = .16, p < .041$
Cognitive process words	$r = .26, p < .001, r^2 = .07$*	$r = .14, p < .096$
Causation words	$r = .13, p < .090$	$r = .12, p < .110$
Insight words	$r = .16, p < .040$	$r = .03, p < .772$
Discrepancy words	$r = .19, p < .013, r^2 = .04$*	$r = .05, p < .513$
Inhibition words	$r = .05, p < .560$	$r = .01, p < .899$
Tentative words	$r = .09, p < .239$	$r = .23, p < .003, r^2 = .05$*
Certainty words	$r = .18, p < .020, r^2 = .03$*	$r = .09, p < .228$

Note.—*Significant correlation ($\alpha = 0.02$).

to level that was itself significantly related to age, and the only trend that still persisted was the use of words longer than six letters. The number of tentative words (e.g., "maybe," "perhaps," "guess"), however, was significantly correlated with age, although it was not significantly correlated with level. In general, then, level appeared to be more heavily correlated with the 10 markers of linguistic sophistication than was chronological age. The implication of this finding was, as we had hoped, that level seemed to be a better predictor of cognitive and linguistic complexity than was the rough proxy of age.

To further examine this association, and the mean differences in cognitive complexity between each of the levels, a MANOVA with the 10 marker variables as dependent variables and level classification as the between factor was found to be significant (Wilk's $\Lambda = 0.447$, $F(40, 574.43) = 3.398$, $p < 0.0005$, partial $\eta^2 = 0.182$). Follow-up ANOVAs found significance for word count ($F(4, 160) = 26.313$, $p < 0.0005$, partial $\eta^2 = 0.397$), words per sentence ($F(4, 160) = 7.066$, $p < 0.0005$, partial $\eta^2 = 0.150$), words more than six letters long ($F(4, 160) = 2.480$, $p = 0.046$, partial $\eta^2 = 0.058$), cognitive process words ($F(4, 160) = 5.358$, $p < 0.0005$, partial $\eta^2 = 0.118$), and causation words ($F(4, 160) = 2.927$, $p = 0.023$, partial $\eta^2 = 0.068$). For the most part, results for the individual means were what would be predicted: a steady increase on these five significant variables as the level classification increased. Table 22 lists these values by level.

Taken all together, these findings also went some important distance toward demonstrating that the Narrative and Essentialism self-continuity warranting strategies that so clearly set Native and non-Native adolescents apart represented distinct but linguistically equivalent forms of self-

TABLE 22

MEAN SCORES AND STANDARD DEVIATIONS FOR MEASURES OF LINGUISTIC COMPLEXITY BY PERSONAL PERSISTENCE LEVEL ASSIGNMENT

Variable	Mean Score (SD)				
	Level 1	Level 2	Level 3	Level 4	Level 5
Word count	423.90	532.25	867.24	1619.96	2877.50
	(243.41)	(285.77)	(554.91)	(1009.03)	(442.95)
Words per sentence	6.92	10.37	11.58	13.71	16.79
	(3.22)	(6.72)	(6.11)	(4.69)	(3.29)
Words >6 letters	10.44	12.05	11.58	11.99	12.01
	(2.20)	(2.46)	(2.20)	(1.58)	(1.09)
Cognitive process words	6.87	8.12	8.84	8.77	10.13
	(2.70)	(3.30)	(2.03)	(1.62)	(0.77)
Causation words	1.06	1.51	1.54	1.36	1.77
	(0.85)	(0.92)	(0.68)	(0.53)	(0.39)

understanding, both of which showed strong relations with age and available measures of cognitive and linguistic complexity.

Measures of Cultural Commitment and Forms of Self-Understanding

In addition to warding off possible attempts to reductively reinterpret our data as some artifact of cognitive or linguistic complexity, we were also interested in discounting other possible patterns of superficial differences that might be used to explain away what we believed was a much deeper-seated understanding of the self. One such potential discounting possibility was the prospect that Narrative and Essentialist strategies, as we measured them, were simply proxies of some other more tried-and-true, and so presumably better understood, measure of self-concept. Although we have argued (see chapter III) that our participants' self-continuity warranting strategies demark more of a "process" variable than anything they might be explicitly aware of or able to be self-evaluative toward, we were compelled for conceptual reasons to put this assumption to some sort of test. For this reason, and as a way of examining this discounting strategy, a subsample of the First Nations youth who completed our Personal Persistence Interview ($N = 48$, mean age = 16.4 years), as well as other First Nations youth ($N = 94$, mean age = 16.3 years) from the same communities, were also asked to complete a battery of measures meant to assess different and more explicit or objective dimensions of their thinking about the self, and their relations to their culture. By comparing Narrativists and Essentialists on these various scales, we intended to specifically counter the possible criticisms that these ways of thinking about the self are either simply artifacts of certain idiosyncratic ways of characterizing one's self-attributes, or some global difference in the ability of these two groups to employ internal trait descriptions or otherwise more subjectively oriented psychological terms that makes Narrativists and Essentialists only appear to be different in their approaches to problems of personal persistence. As a means of pursuing these possibilities, subsamples of our participants were administered the *Twenty Statements Test* (TST; Kuhn & McPartland, 1954), Singelis' (1994) questionnaire for assessing individuals' Independent and Interdependent self-construals, and Dweck's (2000) *Implicit Theories of Personality Scale*.

Self-Understanding: "The Twenty Statements Test"

To address the possibility that Narrativists were categorized on the basis of some general absence of the trait concepts or subjective psychological terms so central to most Essentialist forms of reasoning, we presented a subsample of First Nations adolescents with the TST.

The TST is an instrument meant to bring to the surface participants' most salient self-descriptions, and is generally considered a useful tool for examining the potential differences in self-concept among men and women or across cultures (Bochner, 1994; Dhawan, Roseman, Naidu, Thapa, & Rettek, 1995; Triandis, 1989; Verkuyten, 1989). The measure itself amounts to little more than a list of 20 sentence stems, all beginning with the phrase "I am...." Participants are left with the job of finishing these incomplete phrases in whatever ways they deem fit.

Although there is some track record of using the TST in cross-cultural research (e.g., Bochner, 1994; Ip & Bond, 1995; Kitayama & Marcus, 1994; Watkins et al., 1998; Watkins & Regmi, 1996), little in the way of agreement exists concerning the best method for scoring participants' responses. There are several scoring systems, allowing anywhere from just 2 to 59 possible response categories—a range that some regard as bounded only by the whims of the researcher (Wells & Marwell, 1976). Many have used the traditional "A-B-C-D" method developed by Kuhn and McPartland (1954) and have extended or retailored it for use with various specialized study populations. This framework for grouping responses into categories of physical (A), social (B), attributive (C), and global (D) statements about the self, although popular, seemed ill suited for our interests, in large part because it has been criticized for its reliance on predominantly "Western" categories, as well as because of the emphasis it places on "decontextualized" accounts of the self. In the face of these problems, the strategy we eventually adopted was that of Watkins et al. (1998), a scoring scheme recently conceived for use in a cross-cultural context and that seemed especially well suited for our present purpose.

Altogether then, the scoring categories we employed were, after Watkins et al. (1998), as follows:

Idiocentric: Statements about personal qualities, attitudes, beliefs, states, and traits that *do not* relate to other people (e.g., I am intelligent, I am happy).

Large group: Statements about large group memberships (where many people are involved), demographic characteristics, and large groups with which people share a common fate (e.g., I am a girl, I am a basketball player).

Small group: As above but for small groups, usually the family is involved (e.g., I am a husband, I am a mother).

Allocentric: Statements about interdependence, friendship, responsiveness to others, or sensitivity to how others perceive you (e.g., I am sociable, I am a person who helps others).

Nearly half (i.e., 45%) of the 91 TST respondents were able to generate 15 or more sentence stems, but many found it difficult to attain the 20 requested. Previous research (Watkins, Yau, Dahlin, & Wondimu, 1997) has addressed this problem, however, and found that, when the current scoring strategy is used, differences in the proportions of the four coding categories for respondents are rare when participants are able to complete at least 7 sentences. Nearly 90% of our sample was able to comply with this reduced production criterion. The mean number of responses, then, was 13.4 ($SD = 5.52$), and ranged from 3 to 20.

Although there were some differences in the scoring profiles for the two Native communities tested, and for the males and females in our sample, there were no statistically significant differences in the TST scores for Narrativists and Essentialists, Wilk's $\Lambda = 0.963$, $F(4, 43) = 0.411$, $p = 0.800$. Most important, these results suggested that Narrativists and Essentialists generated roughly the same sorts of descriptive statements about themselves, even when it came to idiocentric and allocentric claims having to do with either subjective psychological traits or other-oriented characteristics. It hardly seemed the case, then, as some might suggest, that Narrativists are simply those more inclined to talk about others, while Essentialists speak primarily about themselves and the details of their interpsychic lives.

Independent and Interdependent Self-Contruals

Finally, because the dimensions of idiocentrism and allocentrism, in particular, have been measured in other and more explicit ways in the literature (e.g., Markus & Kitayama, 1991), and because we wanted to take still further confirmatory steps toward our claim that Narrativists and Essentialists are not simply using some different "me versus them" forms of speech, we borrowed Singelis' (1994) widely used questionnaire for assessing individuals' independent and interdependent self-construals. In many ways, Singelis' measure parallels the scoring dimensions we extracted from our sample using the TST. Unlike the TST, however, respondents to Singelis' Self-Construal Scale (SCS) are not left to their own devices in coming up with statements about themselves, a task demand that has raised concerns about the TST's use with younger participants and with individuals from non-Western cultures (Watkins et al., 1997), who are said to often be more reluctant to volunteer personal information. Rather, the SCS consists of 24 generic self-descriptions with which respondents either agree or disagree on a 7-point scale. The items of the scale have been factor-analyzed into the two groups of statements: independent and interdependent descriptions. The independent category, much like the idiocentric dimension of the TST, has to do with an understanding of the self that is bounded, unitary, and stable. Such a self-concept is thought to be reflected in statements that emphasize internal states, feelings, and traits, and that stress issues of uniqueness or standing out, as well as promoting one's personal goals. Examples include: "I am comfortable being singled out for praise or rewards" and "My personal identity independent of others is important to me." By contrast, the interdependent category, much like the allocentric dimension of the TST, deals with statements that reflect a flexible and variable self. Here the emphasis is on external or public features of the self such as roles and relationships, as well as on matters dealing with fitting in and finding one's proper place in groups. Statements said to reflect this more interdependent factor include: "It is important for me to maintain harmony within my group," "My happiness depends on the happiness of those around me," and "I respect people who are modest about themselves."

What is of potential interest in our findings from the SCS was that, just as with the Twenty Statements Test, no significant differences emerged in our Native sample. The Urban Native and Rural Native youth did not differ on either of Singelis' independent or interdependent scales, Wilk's $\Lambda = 0.988$, $F(2, 90) = 0.551$, $p = 0.579$. In addition, all of the Native youth scored as high on the independent scale as they did on the interdependent scale, $F(1, 91) = 1.861$, $p = 0.176$. Even in a culture that is alleged to be more collectivistic or relational or otherwise group-oriented, the Native adolescents we interviewed understood themselves in both independent and interdependent terms, and did so to an extent that ruled out any prospect that they thought of these categories as mutually exclusive. More important—and this was the point of adopting the measure in the first place—Narrativists and Essentialists did not differ in their responses on the SCS, allowing us to say with justifiable confidence that the real difference between them was not merely some special readiness on the part of Narrativists to see themselves in "collectivist" terms while Essentialists were more inclined to dwell on their own individuality.

Implicit Theories of Personality

So far we have been happy to report a series of null results to our questions of how Narrativists and Essentialists go about responding to more or less direct measures of their own personal self-concept. More specifically, our findings with the TST and SCS have provided us greater license to conclude that differences in how Narrativists and Essentialists reason about matters of self-continuity really are distinct from, and irreducible to, the more mundane matters of how they talk about themselves or describe their own personal ways of being in the world. Still, what these results do *not* allow us to conclude, at least not directly, is just how Narrativists and Essentialists conceive of personality or character change in some more global or abstract sense apart from their own particular self-concepts. The aim of finding some assessment tool that would tackle this question of personality understanding head on, and that might co-vary with our own measure of self-continuity, was the impetus behind our use of Dweck's (2000) 6-item inventory for measuring individuals' "implicit theories" of personality. Dweck's measure, much like our own, is argued to assess aspects of the self more akin to James's subjective or implicit "I" than to objective "Me" variables associated with self-concept measures like the TST or SCS. Depending on how strongly respondents agreed or disagreed on a 7-point scale to such statements as "Your personality is a part of you that you can't change very much" or "No matter who you are or how you act, you can always change your ways," our sample was scored as either reflecting an altogether "process" orientation, and so a view of personality that allowed for relatively easy change, or a more static "entity" orientation according to which personality is seen as made up of enduring traits that withstand change. Dweck's particular interpretation of these two views, although conceived (and measured) in ways quite different from our own, nevertheless provided a possible parallel to our own strategies for differentiating Essentialists' and Narrativists' responses to questions of self-continuity.

As it turns out, and despite being hampered by a lack of power in our analyses, the anticipated pattern of covariation did emerge as a strong trend (i.e., $\chi^2(1) = 3.59, p = .058$). Specifically, of the small group of Essentialists in our subsample of Native youths ($N = 8$), six, or 75%, fell below the mean on Dweck's scale, indicating that they held an entity view of personality. Just the opposite was true for the 39 Narrativists: 62% were above Dweck's mean score, indicating that they held a more process view of personality. Although some caution must be shown in interpreting these thin results, we take these findings as another step toward validating our Narrativist and Essentialist coding strategies, and demonstrating the differences between these two ways of understanding personal persistence.

Measuring Ethnic Identification

Having succeeded in ruling out the several reductive possibilities discussed above, we were left with one final but critical step. Our main finding, the one we have been defending against potential critiques by the more reductively inclined—the finding that most Native youth were Narrativists and most non-Native youth were Essentialists—and our repeated assertion that the source of this difference can be found in their respective cultural backgrounds, failed to directly address that small rump group of participants who behaved in "countercultural" ways. That is, even though our categorical expectations were not met in every instance, we were under an obligation to offer some explanation for the fact that a nontrivial number of our observations fell into the "wrong" cells. That is, some of our Native respondents did adopt Essentialist ways and some of our non-Native participants responded in Narrative ways. It was possible, therefore, that the young people in our Native sample who employed warranting strategies that were more common in the mainstream culture were, perhaps, proportionally less invested in their own culture of origin. It seemed important, therefore, to take some measure of the possibility that differences in the depth or focus on their identification with First Nations culture would predict Native participants' choice of warranting strategies. What was obviously required was some measure of ethnic identification appropriate for use with our Native sample.

Without attempting anything that could legitimately pass for a real review, we mean only to point out for the benefit of those unfamiliar with this literature that the art of measuring (by way of questionnaires) the degree to which individuals value or practice the distinguishing details of what they take to be their "heritage culture" could be most charitably thought of as being "still in its infancy." The usual rough-hewn practice has been to simply ask, in some direct fashion, whether respondents actually participate, or otherwise like or dislike, the usual details (i.e., food, music, dances, clothing, etc.) commonly associated with their own and other ethnic groups. What is easily lost in this perhaps unrealistically hopeful approach is any serious prospect of distinguishing between what people will lay claim to and what they really think or do, a problem of special salience in First Nations communities where the political demands of the "pan-Indian" movement and the special premium currently placed on anything "traditional" requires taking every self-proclamation in favor of Native ways with a large grain of salt. Still, there is a collection of usual ways to go about measuring ethnic identity, and we patched together four of the most widely used and psychometrically well-tutored measures of ethnic identity currently available and gave them to our samples of Urban and Rural Native youth. By design, such measures of ethnic identification were judged inappropriate for use with our non-Native sample.

The questionnaire was presented to 48 of the Native participants who had previously completed the Personal Persistence Interview. The various measures that went into our initial 130-item Ethnic Identification questionnaire were:

1. Vancouver Index of Acculturation (VIA; Ryder et al., 2000), a self-report instrument that assesses several domains relevant to acculturation, including values, social relationships, and adherence to traditions.

2. Ward and Rana-Deuba's (1999) Acculturation Index, which assesses two dimensions (host and co-national identification) and four modes (integration, separation, marginalization, and assimilation) of acculturation.

3. Phinney's (1992) Multigroup Ethnic Identity Measure (MEIM), a questionnaire measure designed for use across diverse ethnic groups.

4. Zygmuntowiscz et al.'s (2000) Values Orientation Scale, a version of an earlier measure by Szapocnik et al. (1978) that has been specifically adapted to assess acculturation in First Nations adolescents.

Pursued by concerns that in our bid for inclusiveness we had ended up with more items than subjects, two after-the-fact steps were taken to somewhat whittle down, for the purposes of analyses, the length of this questionnaire. This was done in two ways. The first and easiest was to simply adopt the Vancouver Index of Acculturation (a recently normed measure that was built on the back of the other three measures already included) as the best of what is available. The other was to regard the full complement of these four published measures as one overly ambitious item pool, and to proceed to drop items with little variance, to weed out more or less semantically identical items, and to choose among items that were so highly correlated as to be statistically redundant. The 30-item scale arrived at in this way was then factor-analyzed, resulting in two factors: one marked a preference for all things Native, the other indicated an affinity for things non-Native.

In the end, this attempt to understand why some Native youth parted company with the majority of their fellows and choose Essentialism largely failed. In part, we were hampered from the start by a lack of statistical power brought on not just by our small sample size (48), but more so by the low number of Native youth classified as Essentialist. That problem we could have solved. What we should (in hindsight) have been better prepared for was the extent to whichthe Native youth (Narrative and Essentialist alike) effectively pounced on many items from the "Native" side of our scale. That is, in the response style, if not in the minds of these Native participants, all things Native were clearly said to be better than almost anything imaginable. Programs to promote Native pride clearly appear to be working—working so well, in fact, that there was little if any real variance in our measures of ethnic identification. Narrative or Essentialist, Native youth consistently claimed to prefer and value all things Native.

SUMMARY OF RESULTS

Whatever else might divide the young persons who made up our Native and non-Native groups, they were not different in terms of age or in the ratio of males to females. There was also no evidence to suggest that our interview techniques were beyond the ability of any but a fraction of our young participants, or that our choice of interview materials or the medium in which those materials were presented had any differential effect on participants from any one community or cultural group. There is strong evidence, however, that our Personal Persistence Interview yielded data that can be reliably coded to generate Track and Level classifications for each participant. Track (or type) of reasoning was not related to age or to gender, but was strongly associated with cultural background: Native youth predominantly employed Narrative arguments and non-Native youth predominantly employed Essentialist arguments. The level of sophistication of such arguments was not, however, related to cultural background or gender, but was, as expected, related to age. Our longitudinal data showed that adopting either a Narrative or Essentialist approach to the problem of personal persistence was stable across a two-year interval, but, predictably, Level was not—a finding indicating that the type of reasoning one employs is a more or less persistent strategy of thought about matters of self-continuity, whereas the complexity of such thoughts can and does often grow over the course of development.

Because of the special conceptual significance that we attached to observed cultural differences with respect to Track, we wanted to be especially certain that this distinction was not the result of background differences in linguistic or cognitive sophistication that might be imagined to characterize our groups, or that it was not simply the product of differing but extracurricular ways of construing or understanding the concepts of self or personality change. In each case, our analyses provided strong reassurance. Essentialists and Narrativists do not differ in the extent to which they endorse idiocentric and allocentric statements, or independent and interdependent conceptions of identity. They do show a tendency to differ, however, and in just the way one would predict: in their implicit theories of personality, with Narrativists championing personality change and Essentialists favoring enduring immutable traits. It also might have been the case (but was not) that the roots of this cultural difference were to be found in differing levels of commitment to one's cultural group. That is, it might have been that a narrative or relational way of speaking was somehow seen by our Native participants as particularly "Indian" and, therefore, the "right" way of speaking to non-Native researchers regardless of one's real thoughts about personal persistence or anything else. If that were true, one would expect to find Native Narrativists to be more strongly committed to First Nations culture than Native Essentialists. Our data do not show that. Instead, though the Native youth in our sample were (on the whole) strongly committed to the value of their cultural heritage, multiple measures of ethnic identification failed to distinguish Narrativists from Essentialists in this regard. The clear conclusion supported by all of these analyses was that culture is very strongly associated with whether one adopts a Narrative and Essentialist strategy for resolving the paradox of personal persistence and change.

VII. CONCLUSIONS

Evidence of the sort we have brought out in this *Monograph* touches not only on heartfelt matters about which many people have strong and entrenched opinions but also on prior research claims and hard-won theoretical positions that are not always consistent with our own. We recognize that others have made serious personal and professional investments in alternative claims and that it would profit them to assimilate our findings to their own ends. As such, the opportunities for us to be misinterpreted or misunderstood are many. We, of course, are just as eager to be understood as saying just what we mean, and to avoid having our points dulled by being forced into shapes for which they were not designed. What follows, then, is our final effort to say bluntly what we mean, and to ward off at least some of the more obvious ways in which we might be most easily misunderstood. Although there is perhaps, somewhere, a still longer list of misleading leap-to-mind conclusions to which our working distinction between Narrative and Essentialist self-continuity warranting strategies might be misapplied, the following Top Five list will do for a start.

On Why Narrativity Is Not the Logical Opposite or Negative Co-Relative of Essentialism

First, Narrativity and Essentialism are not meant as candidates for becoming merely the latest in a seemingly endless series of social science dichotomies intended to neatly pigeonhole people into one or the other of two watertight compartments. They are not intended as the two halves of anything; nonetheless, intended or not, it is easy enough to see how our work might promote such a reading. Throughout this *Monograph*, we have contrasted Essentialist and Narrative strategies at least a hundred times. Who wouldn't feel well within their rights in imagining that we were dichotomizers after all, plainly convicted out of our own mouths. Our problem—hopefully not entirely of our own making—is that our research has uncovered just these two (as opposed to three or six) self-continuity warranting strategies, and "two," in the individual differences game, is an unlucky number, in large part because of the messy "residue of dichotomizing" (Oyserman, Coon, & Kemmelmeier, 2002) it regularly gives off. Particularly as they bear on the task of theorizing about whole cultures and so are easily imagined to serve as "pillars of human life" (Bakan, 1966), such broad bivalent taxonomies (e.g., agentic vs. communal; egocentric vs. sociocentric; rights-based vs. duty-based; individualistic vs. ensembled, or holistic, or collectivistic) typically work to overlook complexities within cultures and within social groups (Overton, 1998) and, as Kagitcibasi (1996) has shown, regularly fail to capture much of what is happening in the identity development of people, especially Third World people. Worse still, and perhaps because they traffic so heavily in matters of shared beliefs and values, such bare-bones, either-or conjunctions easily become propagandized, and they have tended to serve as shorthand political slogans for all things modern and Western as opposed to things traditional and non-Western. Little wonder then that we worry over whether, by having identified Essentialist and Narrative self-continuity warranting practices as the only apparent games in town, we may have inadvertently played into the hands of dichotomizers who automatically suppose that every matter of psychological import naturally yields two (and only two) logically oppositional alternatives.

We hope, for reasons we have already worked to make clear, that Essentialist and Narrative practices are not at all like that. Essentialism is decidedly *not*, in our view, the negative co-relative of Narrative approaches to personal persistence, nor is one of these practices the logical reciprocal or the inverse of the other, and both together do not somehow logically exhaust the set of potentially workable ways of thinking about self-continuity in time. Most familiar social science dichotomies (e.g., agentic vs. communal societies) reference what are meant to be "exclusive unions" and admit numerically distinct parts (Grene, 1988), parts that do not share the same ontological status and stand instead in relations that are of an exclusively empirical nature (e.g., cause-effect; antecedent-consequent). Such parts are distinct and do not share the same ontological identity. Narrative and Essentialist strategies, however—whether viewed at the individual or group level—are not like that. Instead, they form "inclusive unions" in which the different so-called parts or facets are not "numerically distinct differences in existence, but rather differences in the mode of manifestation of what is effectively the same existence" (Chandler, 1991, p. 13). In this sense, Narrative and Essentialist warranting practices, like the selves and cultures that host them, are not merely empirically related as discrete or separate entities might be, rather they are alternative manifestations of one and the same thing. In short, not everything of which there are only two available instances automatically amounts to logical opposites or dichotomies, including Essentialist and Narrative solutions to the problem of personal persistence.

Avoiding the Individualism-Collectivism Antinomy

Second, having made the case that our distinction between Essentialist and Narrative self-continuity warranting strategies is not simply one more attempt to divide the world into two contrary and logically opposite pictures without remainder, we feel compelled to try to similarly ward off the prospect that these strategies might also be mistakenly viewed as somehow subsumable under the seemingly horizonless and oversubscribed "individualism versus collectivism" antinomy. The temptation to collapse these two differently conceived accounting schemes is clearly strong. After all, couldn't "essences" be easily read as just the sort of thing naturally assumed to hide out in the secret hearts of individuals, just as "narratives," which necessarily imply listeners as well as narrators, would seem to automatically implicate collectives? Why, given all of this, should we not simply relax and allow our ideas to be assimilated into the ubiquitous distinction between all things *Individualistic* as opposed to *Collectivistic*. Attractive though this might appear to some, giving into any such a temptation would, in our own "collective" judgment, be a serious mistake.

Our aversion to the prospect of seeing anything else (including our own Essentialist/Narrative distinction) reduced to the status of a mere footnote on the larger-than-life Individualism/Collectivism page is not an aversion particular to ourselves. Of late, critics of this popular distinction appear to be winning new converts on an almost daily basis, and winning them in some of the most unlikely places (e.g., Kitayama, 2002; Miller, 2002). Still, such fault-finding is rather new, and it would be unwise to prematurely discount the strength of the gravitational force that operates to draw everything in its path into the popular Individualism/Collectivism orbit. As Triandis (1989) has pointed out, individualism-collectivism has, for a very long time, been "the single most important dimension of cultural differences in social behavior," so important, in fact, that Kagitcibasi (1996) has "identified the 1980s as the decade of individualism-collectivism" (Hermans & Kempen, 1998, p. 1112). Nor, according to Lonner and Adamopoulos (1997), does this trend show any real signs of abating. In short, until very recently and with very few exceptions (Turiel, 2002; Turiel & Wainryb, 1994), one dared speak only in the most reverential terms about the so-called "I/C" distinction.

All of that, of course, was then. *Now*—where "now" refers to a specious present whose width can still be measured in months—enthusiasm for the individualism-collectivism dichotomy is increasingly seen to be fading, due in no small part to rather recent critiques by some of its most ardent former admirers (e.g., Kitayama, 2002; Miller, 2002; Oyserman et al., 2002). Increasingly, contributors to this literature (e.g., Church, 2000; Kagitcibasi, 1996; Matsumoto, 1999) have begun to view attempts to characterize whole cultures or individuals in terms of broad cultural dichotomies (e.g., duty-based vs. rights-based, independent vs. interdependent; egocentric vs. sociocentric, individualistic vs. collectivistic) as both crude and misleading.

The list of reasons currently being given in support of this new disaffection is both long and varied. Highly ranked among the unflattering things currently being said behind the back of the I/C distinction is that, rather than working as a binary choice, these alternatives are increasingly understood as common parts of a single control system (Kitayama, 2002), parts that "differ primarily in the likelihood that [they] will be activated" in one cultural context or another (Oyserman et al., 2002, p. 115). In addition to being increasingly discounted as a false dichotomy (Miller, 2002), the I/C distinction is also repeatedly faulted for (a) focusing too exclusively on attitudes and values at the expense of more dynamic practices and associated mental processes (D'Andrade, 2001; Kitayama, 2002); (b) depending on survey methods that assess only declarative self-knowledge, and inevitably fail to make contact with the more tacit procedural competencies that form the core of culture (Bond, 2002; Fiske, 2002); and (c) coming "dangerously close to minimizing individual agency in favor of cultural determinism" (Gjerde & Onishi, 2000, p. 219). Because the Individualism and Collectivism dichotomy appears to be in serious decline, and because efforts to breathe new life back into it appear to involve making it look increasingly like our own more inclusive and procedurally oriented distinction between Narrative and Essentialist approaches to the self, we respectfully decline the invitation to be among the last aboard the sinking ship of Individualism-Collectivism.

On Committing the Psychologist's Fallacy and Getting Away With It

Although many would see it as missing the larger point, few would dispute the right of social scientists to set about studying the internal dynamics of individual selves. Nor would many object to an enterprise devoted to working out how whole communities, or whole cultures, are best imagined to differ from one another in their collective ways of viewing selves in time. But a really serious mistake, it has generally been alleged, would arise if the same person or research team were to seriously envision simultaneously doing both. One important part of what we hope you will be taking away from this *Monograph* is that the procedural means by which young persons undertake to warrant their own convictions about personal persistence do not lend themselves to being best understood in the recommended serial fashion had in mind by such critics.

Our own data suggest, instead, that young people's temporally vectored conceptions of themselves and others are neither the exclusive province of matters entirely internal to themselves, nor are they the exclusive consequence of socially constructed (and so culturally variable) practices already in place in their communities. Rather, our findings would suggest, not only is it the case that neither of these antinomous options seem true on their face, but that even the decision to put the matter in these split, either-or terms is itself a mistake. Instead, it would appear from the evidence we have brought forward that the task of working out what it could possibly mean to have or be a self needs to be viewed as existing within a problem space that occupies at least three different levels of problem description (see Chandler et al., 2000; Chandler & Sokol, in press). At the most abstract of these levels (what Marr, 1982, calls the "computational" or "design" level), every individual and every culture must, on pain of otherwise failing to satisfy those minimal design requirements necessary for the maintenance of any social or moral order whatsoever, include some computational means of solving the universal problem of sameness within difference, and thus allowing both individuals and whole communities to understand themselves as somehow continuous in the face of inevitable personal and cultural change. Importantly, however, nothing about such claims in favor of the existence of transcultural commonalities needs or ought to be seen as in any way impugning the evident fact that different cultural groups make available to their members culturally contingent default strategies for constructing and preserving the self in time. Nor is it, our data would suggest, ever the case that any two young people—whatever their public and private circumstance—need actually end up instrumenting their developmental and cultural and even, perhaps, human obligations to persistence by actually proceeding in precisely the same way. Without careful attention to the different levels of problem description on which such claims operate, all of those (ourselves included) who aim to examine issues of identity development at both the individual and cultural level risk having their claims once again hijacked by those whose "split" polemic (Overton, 1998) threatens to return us to that dichotomized place where the only permissible question is "which one?"

On Why Essentialism and Narrativity Are Not Simply Code for the West Versus Everyone Else

As Kagitcibasi pointed out, "individualism is [commonly] seen as akin to modernity and is associated with modern values [while] collectivism is seen to embody traditional, conservative ideology" (1996, p. 63), all of which works to suspiciously align those who traffic in such constructs with those less reputable champions of persistent neocolonialist practices who seek to naturalize and legitimize their actions by passing them off as well-intended efforts to bring the Third and Fourth Worlds into the 21st century. What Third and Fourth World peoples actually believed to be true about themselves prior to contact is, of course, largely speculation. What is not so much in doubt is that by portraying one's own group as in good equilibrium it is often possible to minimize state interference and maximize local autonomy. Consequently, the job of calculating the real extent to which indigenous peoples have become socialized into actually imagining themselves to be somehow more collectivist and harmonious than their colonizers, and sorting all of this out from the degree to which such forms of self-presentation are truly heartfelt as opposed to strategically political and counterhegemonic, is a Solomon-like exercise for which social-science training typically leaves one poorly prepared. Wherever the cut is eventually made, it is already clear enough that simply accepting, on its face, continuing easy talk about individualism and collectivism demands a kind of innocence that all but the most insular have long since lost. There are, by contrast, good reasons to suppose that the distinction between Narrative and Essentialist approaches to the problem of personal persistence is not like that.

First, such category assignments were made, not by our respondents themselves, but by coders who worked behind the scenes carefully summing up records of earlier practices and procedures put to use by our respondents as they attempted to negotiate problems about sameness in the face of change. As such, few if any of the young participants in our studies had any declarative or well semanticized knowledge of their own self-continuity warranting practices, and so could not make use of such information for the purposes of impression management if they tried.

Second, what our assessment procedures were meant to measure was not some hidden competence that occurs, or is better measured, in some more than in others. We have every reason to believe—and some good empirical reasons to know—that most (perhaps all) of the participants in our research were "capable" of answering in either a Narrative or Essentialist voice. Consequently, what we took ourselves to be measuring, and what we believed culture and development was shaping was not ability but accessibility and the tendency for young persons socialized in different ways to employ different default strategies to problems of personal persistence.

On the Merits and Demerits of Narrative and Essentialist Strategies

Fifth and finally, in this list of cautionary tales, is our concern that our work not be somehow swept into that evaluative framework of understanding according to which it is imagined possible to determine whether "some cultures are linked to higher stages of development than are others" (Oyserman et al., 2002, p. 1110). It is in no way our point to attempt to argue that either Narrative or Essentialist practices are inherently more adequate than the other, or to imagine that there is some neutral scale of values on which these different strategies can be weighed. That is, although we take it that there is a universal obligation on us all to compute some workable self-continuity warranting strategy, there are no principled grounds for deciding in the abstract how the contrastive heuristics represented by Narrative and Essentialist solutions will fare in the face of whatever adversities blind circumstance might throw into one's personal or collective path. Durkheim (1897/1952), for example, made a compelling case that when "individuals sense that their own norms and values are no longer relevant, and ... when people are forced to respond to conditions that they have little or no ability to control" (Clayer & Czechowicz, 1991, p. 685), then a sense of anomie and elevated suicide rates regularly follow. It is also equally possible to imagine that, especially during periods of rapid cultural change, Essentialism, though not without some alienating consequences of its own, could sometimes succeed in carrying one away from the situationally troubled surface and toward some quieter, more subterranean pool of abstraction where the core of one's self is alleged to be found. What seems impossible to imagine, however, is that a Narrative strategy (or perhaps any strategy) could still be made to work if, after millenia of success, one's cultural practices were criminalized and systemically deconstructed through government-sponsored programs of cultural assimilation, that there would still seem enough in the way of future prospects and of a past to call one's own to warrant much in the way of a commitment to go on living.

Summary

Having discussed over the last several pages a handful of ways in which our work might be (perhaps even lends itself to being) misinterpreted, and having struggled to make ourselves better understood, what remains to be said by way of simple summary can be wrapped up small, and delivered as five succinct points.

First, in chapters I and II, a conceptual case was made that recourse to some form of self-understanding capable of preserving a sense of personal and cultural persistence is an identity-conferring obligation that must be satisfied if there is to be any followable meaning to personal and social life, and so is presumably common to all human cultures.

Second, in chapter III, we presented the details of a descriptive framework used in the forging of methods and procedures that could be, and were, used to mark the fact that young people ordinarily exercise different understandings of the grounds for their own personal persistence as they move through the usual weigh-stations that mark the course of their own conceptual and identity development. The upshot of these efforts was a typology, and associated scoring scheme, that parsed what young people actually do say on the subject of personal persistence into what we came to call Narrative and Essentialist self-continuity warranting strategies: age-graded, cognitively sanctioned strategies available for exploitation in accomplishing the performative task of justifying self-sameness in the face of inevitable change.

Third, and in chapter IV, we turned to a special population of seriously suicidal adolescents as a way of testing, and then substantiating, the strongly theory-driven expectation that those who fail to successfully sustain some self-continuity warranting strategies suffer, as a natural consequence, a loss of connectedness to their own future, and are thereby placed at special risk for suicide.

Fourth, we went on in chapter V to explore the hypothesis that individual and cultural continuity are strongly linked. We did this by mounting what proved to be a strong demonstration that First Nations communities that succeed in taking steps to preserve their heritage culture and to recover some measure of control over the institutions governing their own collective future are also dramatically more successful in insulating their own children against the risks of suicide

Fifth and finally, chapter VI was given over to a demonstration that different cultures (in this case the Canadian cultural mainstream and selected First Nations communities) serve to promote different approaches to the problem of personal persistence, with essentialist strategies more favored among those young persons who are the direct inheritors of a "modern" Euro-American tradition, and narrative means of warranting their own and others' self-continuity chosen more often by Aboriginal adolescents.

Taken altogether, these new lines of evidence go some distance toward making the case that, though the young members of at least these several distinct communities all struggle to cope with common questions posed by the shared experience of being a self awash in the flux of time, the answers that they provide in attempting to count themselves and others as personally persistent are clearly influenced by a synergistic mix of matters that are now known to include their current place in the course of their own development and the historical or cultural circumstances of their lives. Although perhaps interesting in its own right, the potential importance of this line of evidence is lent a special significance by the fact that the manner in which individual young persons, and even whole communities, manage hard questions concerning their own survival in time has been shown here to contribute to their decision as to whether life is or is not worth living. Such hard to acquire data do not, of course, finally settle any of the classic controversies they are meant to address, but, given the magnitude of the personal and cultural problems at which they are aimed, they are perhaps a beginning.

Beginnings, of course, are first steps in undertakings that, so far, have been done only in the least degree. Our own undertaking is naturally of this beginning sort. What we claim to have initiated is a program of empirical research that lays the groundwork for an interlacing network of proven relations that, when closer to completion, will successfully link problems in personal or cultural persistence with youth suicide. Some of these separate links are already forged. Our data show, for example, that (a) young persons who lose the thread of their own personal persistence are at special risk to suicide, (b) that community level rates of suicide among Aboriginal youth are strongly associated with various markers of cultural continuity, and (c) that Aboriginal youth typically undertake to solve problems of personal persistence by relying on what we have termed Narrative strategies that are markedly different from the Essentialist strategies typically practiced by non-Aboriginal youth.

Although each of these empirical links adds to the connectivity of our argument, other nodes and cords in this still loose explanatory network are principally held in place only by strong intuitions and surmise. We argue, for example, that the evident communalities between self-continuity and cultural continuity are more than simply semantic, and that the fact that each serves as a hedge against suicide suggest an entanglement of evidence that goes beyond the mere analogical. We say this, but we cannot yet prove it. Similarly, we have speculated that Narrative solutions to the problem of personal persistence (the solution strategies preferred by 8 out of 10 of the Aboriginal youth), although formally no better or worse than more Essentialist solutions, may be especially vulnerable to organized attempts at cultural deconstruction of the sorts to which Aboriginal peoples and other colonized groups have commonly been subjected. Some support for this hypothesis is provided by the fact that lower rates of youth suicide are evident in those Aboriginal communities that have been especially successful in reclaiming their own past and regaining control over their own future; nevertheless, to discount the possibility that some alternative further fact may also account for these same findings, stronger, less correlational evidence is required. By way of repair, we are currently involved in a more experimental program of intervention/prevention research meant to better test the linkages between community control and harm reduction—an effort that holds the potential of strengthening the existing empirical links between such community-based initiatives and various health-related outcome measures. Similarly, we have already begun to collect evidence concerning suicide rates in other Aboriginal and non-Aboriginal age cohorts as a way of further testing some of our theory-driven claims about the relations between watershed moments in the identity-formation process, problems in personal persistence, and suicidality. Finally, if our claims concerning the importance of sustaining a workable sense of personal persistence are in the running for truth, then those who drop the thread of their own continuity should not only suffer a loss of commitment to their own future well-being but also a counterpart sense of responsibility for their own past. Evidence of the sort we are currently hard about collecting with antisocial youth will hopefully turn this strong intuition into one more in a gathering of still-needed empirical linkages.

APPENDIX: SAMPLE QUESTIONS FROM THE PERSONAL PERSISTENCE INTERVIEW

Jean Valjean

Now that you have heard/read the story of Jean Valjean, I'd like to ask you some questions about him.

To start off, can you just tell me about the main story character Valjean. Describe him the way you would to someone who hasn't heard the story.

Could you say a bit more about what Valjean is like at the *beginning* of the story?

Now let's skip over all the things that happen in the story and just tell me about what Valjean is like at the *end* of the story. How would you describe him then?

At the beginning of the story the central character is called Jean Valjean and at the end he is referred to as Monsieur Madeline. Is Monsieur Madeline really Jean Valjean? The names are different, but are Monsieur Madeline and Jean Valjean one and the same person?

At the beginning of the story the central character is called Jean Valjean and at the end he is referred to as Monsieur Madeline. I noticed that the way you describe Valjean is very different in important ways from the way that you describe Monsieur Madeline.

How was Valjean different at the end of the story than he was at the beginning of the story?

What else might be different about him at the end of the story?

In summary, then, how would you say he has changed?

Given all these important changes, how is it that Valjean and Monsieur Madeline are still one and the same person? Is Monsieur Madeline really Jean Valjean? The names are different, but are Monsieur Madeline and Jean Valjean one and the same person?

You have now told me a lot of things that have changed about Valjean, and listed all the ways that he differs at the end of the story and is unlike the

118

man he was at the beginning. Given all of these changes, what is it that makes Valjean one and the same person throughout the story?

Is Monsieur Madeline really Jean Valjean? The names are different, but are Monsieur Madeline and Jean Valjean one and the same person?

(Assuming that only a list of similarities is offered) You are right—those are important ways that Valjean is the *same*, but the other changes that we talked about still took place. Given all of these important differences, what continues to make Valjean one and the same person? What do you think makes him the same person?

What do you think about Valjean himself? Does Valjean think he is the same person—that is, when he remembers the person he was in the beginning, does he feel that the things that happened then actually happened to the person he now takes himself to be?

How might Valjean explain to someone else that one and the same person could act in all of the different ways that he acted throughout the story?

Self

First, I would like you to describe what sort of person you were five years ago.

If someone didn't know you, what could you say to help them understand the sort of person you were then?

Next, I would like you to describe the sort of person you see yourself as being right now.

It sounds like you have changed in some important ways from the sort of person you were five years ago. What are some of the important changes that have taken place in your life in the last five years or so?

What I now want you to explain—and this is the most important part—is what are the reasons that you think of yourself as the self-same person that you were five years ago. What makes you the same person? Just explain your reasons.

How would you explain all the changes that have taken place in your life? How might you explain to someone else that one and the same person could act in all of the different ways that you have described?

How is it that you have become the person you are right now?

REFERENCES

Aboud, F., & Ruble, D. (1987). Identity constancy in children: Developmental processes and implications. In Honess, T. & Yardley, K. (Eds.) *Self and identity: Perspectives across the lifespan*. New York: Routledge & Kegan Paul.

Bakan, D. (1966). *The duality of human existence*. Chicago: Rand McNally.

Bakhtin, M. (1986). *Speech genres and other late essays*. Austin: University of Texas Press.

Ball, L., & Chandler, M. J. (1989). Identity formation in suicidal and non-suicidal youth: The role of self-continuity. *Development and Psychopathology*, **1**(3), 257–275.

Bandura, A. (1986). From thought to action: Mechanisms of personal agency. *New Zealand Journal of Psychology*, **15**(1), 1–17.

Barclay, C., & Smith, T. (1990). Autobiographical remembering and self-composing. *International Journal of Personal Construct Psychology*, **35**, 59–65.

Baumeister, R. F. (1990). Suicide as escape from self. *Psychological Review*, **97**(1), 90–113.

Beck, H., Weissman, A., Lester, D., & Trexler, L. (1974). The measurement of pessimism: The hopelessness scale. *Journal of Consulting and Clinical Psychology*, **42**, 861–865.

Bell, M. (1990). How primordial is narrative? In Nash, C. (Ed.), *Narrative in culture*. New York: Routledge.

Berzonsky, M. (1993). A constructive view of identity development: People as postpositivist self-theorists. In Kroger, J. (Ed.), *Discussions on ego identity*. Hillsdale, NJ: Erlbaum.

Bierwert, C. (1999). *Brushed by cedar, living by the river: Coast Salish figures of power*. Tucson: University of Arizona Press.

Blasi, A. (1983). The self and cognition. In Lee, B. & Noam, G. (Eds.) *Developmental approaches to the self*. New York: Plenum Press.

Blasi, A., & Milton, K. (1991). The development of the sense of self in adolesence. *Journal of Personality*, **59**, 217–242.

Boas, F. (1911). *The mind of primitive man*. New York: Macmillan.

Bochner, S. (1994). Cross-cultural differences in the self-concept: A test of Hofstede's individualism/collectivism distinction. *Journal of Cross-Cultural Psychology*, **25**, 273–283.

Bond, M. H. (2002). Reclaiming the individual from Hofstede's ecological analysis: A 20-year odyssey: Comment on Oyserman et al. (2002). *Psychological Bulletin*, **128**(1), 73–77.

Borst, S. R., Noam, G. G., & Bartok, J. A. (1991). Adolescent suicidality: A clinical-developmental approach. *Journal of the American Academy of Child and Adolescent Psychiatry*, **32**, 501–508.

British Columbia Vital Statistics Agency. (2001). *Analysis of health statistics for Status Indians in British Columbia: 1991–1999*. Vancouver, B.C.: Author.

Brockelman, P. (1985). *Time and self*. New York: Crossroads.

Brockopp, G. W., & Lester, D. (1970). Time perception in suicidal and non-suicidal individuals. *Crisis Intervention*, **2**, 98–100.

Bruner, J. S. (1986). *Actual minds, possible worlds*. Cambridge, MA: Harvard University Press.

REFERENCES

Bunge, M. (1963). *Causality.* New York: Meridian.

Burd, M. (1994). *Regional analysis of British Columbia's Status Indian population: Birth-related and mortality statistics.* British Columbia: Division of Vital Statistics, British Columbia Ministry of Health and Ministry Responsible for Seniors.

Callinicos, A. (1989). *Against post-modernism.* Oxford: Polity Press.

Campbell, A. (1981). *The sense of well-being in America.* New York: McGraw-Hill.

Car, D. (1986). *Time, narrative, and history.* Bloomington: Indiana University Press.

Carsten, J. (2000). *Cultures of relatedness: New approaches to the study of kinship.* Cambridge, UK: Cambridge University Press.

Cassirer, E. (1923). *Substance and function.* Chicago: Open Court Publishing.

Chandler, M. J. (1991). Alternative readings of the competence-performance relation. In Chandler, M. & Chapman, M. (Eds.) *Criteria for competence: Controversies in the conceptualization and assessment of children's abilities.* Hillsdale, NJ: Erlbaum.

Chandler, M. J. (1994). Self-continuity in suicidal and nonsuicidal adolescents. In Noam, G. & Borst, S. (Eds.) *Children, youth and suicide: Developmental perspectives.* San Francisco: Jossey-Bass.

Chandler, M. J. (1997). Stumping for progress in a post-modern world. In Renninger, K. A. & Amsel, E. (Eds.) *Change and development: Issues of theory, method, and application.* Mahwah, NJ: Erlbaum.

Chandler, M. J. (1999). Foreword. In Scholnick, E. K., Nelson, K., Gelman, S. A. & Miller, P. H. (Eds.) *Conceptual development: Piaget's legacy.* Mahwah, NJ: Erlbaum.

Chandler, M. J. (2000). Surviving time: The persistence of identity in this culture and that. *Culture and Psychology,* **6**(2), 209–231.

Chandler, M. J. (2001). The time of our lives: Self-continuity in Native and non-Native youth. In Reese, H. W. (Ed.), *Advances in child development and behavior: Vol. 28.* New York: Academic Press.

Chandler, M. J., & Ball, L. (1990). Continuity and commitment: A developmental analysis of the identity formation process in suicidal and non-suicidal youth. In Bosma, H. & Jackson, S. (Eds.) *Coping and self-concept in adolescence.* New York: Springer-Verlag.

Chandler, M. J., Boyes, M., Ball, S., & Hala, S. (1986). Continuity and commitment: A developmental analysis of the identity formation process. *The British Columbia Psychologist,* **1**, 17–26.

Chandler, M. J., Boyes, M., Ball, S., & Hala, S. (1987). The conservation of selfhood: Children's changing conceptions of self-continuity. In Honess, T. & Yardley, K. (Eds.) *Self and identity: Perspectives across the life-span.* London: Routledge & Kegan Paul.

Chandler, M. J., & Lalonde, C. E. (1998). Cultural continuity as a hedge against suicide in Canada's First Nations. *Transcultural Psychiatry,* **35**(2), 191–219.

Chandler, M. J., Lalonde, C. E., & Sokol, B. W. (2000). Continuities of selfhood in the face of radical developmental and cultural change. In Nucci, L., Saxe, G. & Turiel, E. (Eds.) *Culture, thought, and development.* Mahwah, NJ: Erlbaum.

Chandler, M. J., & Sokol, B. W. (in press). Level this, level that: The place of culture in the construction of the self. In Raeff, C. & Benson, J. B. (Eds.) *Culture and development: Essays in honor of Ina Uzgiris.* New York: Routledge.

Chisholm, R. M. (1971). On the logic of intentional action. In Binkley, R., Bronaugh, R. & Marras, A. (Eds.) *Agent, action, and reason.* Toronto: University of Toronto Press.

Church, A. T. (2000). Culture and personality: Toward an integrated cultural trait psychology. *Journal of Personality,* **68**, 651–703.

Clayer, J. R., & Czechowicz, A. S. (1991). Suicide by aboriginal people in South Australia: Comparison with suicide deaths in the total urban and rural populations. *Medical Journal of Australia,* **154**, 683–685.

Cohen, L., Davis, R., Miller, T., & Sheppard, M. (2002, May). *Intentional vs. unintentional injury: Bridging the gap.* Paper presented at the 6th World Conference on Injury Prevention and Control, Montreal.

Cole, M. (1999). Culture in development. In Bornstein, M. & Lamb, M. (Eds.) *Developmental psychology: An advanced textbook.* Mahwah, NJ: Erlbaum.

Cooper, M., Corrado, R., Karlberg, A. M., & Pelletier Adams, L. (1992). Aboriginal suicide in British Columbia: An overview. *Canada's Mental Health*, **40**(3), 19–23.

Cornell, S., & Kalt, J. (2000). Where's the glue? Institutional and cultural foundations of American Indian economic development. *Journal of Socio-Economics*, **29**, 443–470.

D'Andrade, R. (2001). A cognitivist's view of the units debate in cultural anthropology. *Cross Cultural Research: The Journal of Comparative Social Science*, **35**(2), 242–257.

Danziger, K. (1997). The historical formation of selves. In Ashmore, R. & Jussin, L. (Eds.) *Self and identity: Fundamental issues.* New York: Oxford University Press.

Deloria Jr., V. (1979). *The metaphysics of modern existence.* San Francisco: Harper & Row.

Dennett, D. C. (1978). *Brainstorms: Philosophical essays on mind and psychology.* Cambridge, MA: MIT Press.

Dennett, D. C. (1987). *The intentional stance.* Cambridge, MA: MIT Press.

Dennett, D. C. (1992). The self as a center of narrative gravity. In Kessel, F. S. & Cole, P. M. (Eds.) *Self and consciousness: Multiple perspectives.* Hillsdale, NJ: Erlbaum.

Derrida, J. (1978). *Writing and difference.* London: Routledge & Kegan Paul.

DeVries, R. (1969). Constancy of generic identity in the years three to six. *Monographs of the Society for Research in Child Development*, **34**(3, Serial No. 127).

Dhawan, N., Roseman, I. J., Naidu, R. K., Thapa, K., & Rettek, S. I. (1995). Self-concepts across two cultures: India and the United States. *Journal of Cross-Cultural Psychology*, **26**, 606–621.

Diamond Goldin, B., & Plewes, A. (1997). *The girl who lived with the bears.* San Diego, CA: Gulliver Books.

Dilthey, W. (1962). *Pattern and meaning in history: Thoughts on history and society.* New York: Harper.

Durkheim, E. (1951). *Suicide: A study in sociology.* Toronto: Collier-McMillan. (Original work published 1897).

Dweck, C. S. (2000). *Self theories: Their role in motivation, personality, and development.* Philadelphia: Psychology Press.

Eakin, P. J. (1999). *How our lives become stories: Making selves.* Ithaca, NY: Cornell University Press.

Elkind, D. (1967). Egocentrism in adolescence. *Child Development*, **38**(4), 1025–1034.

Ennis, J., Barnes, R., & Spenser, J. (1985). Management of the repeatedly suicidal patient. *Canadian Journal of Psychiatry*, **30**, 535–538.

Erikson, E. J. (1968). *Identity: Youth and crisis.* New York: W. W. Norton.

Fiske, P. A. (2002). Using individualism and collectivism to compare culture—A critique of the validity and measurement of the constructs: Comment on Oyserman et al. (2002). *Psychological Bulletin*, **128**(1), 78–88.

Flanagan, O. (1996). *Self expressions: Mind, morals and the meaning of life.* New York: Oxford University Press.

Forster, E. M. (1954). *Aspects of the novel.* New York: Harcourt, Brace, & World. (Originally published 1927).

Fraisse, P. (1963). *The psychology of time.* New York: Harper & Row.

Freeman, M. (1984). History, narrative, and life-span developmental knowledge. *Human Development*, **27**, 1–19.

Fromm, E. (1970). *The crisis of psychoanalysis.* New York: Holt, Rinehart, & Winston.

Gallagher, S. (1998). *The inordinance of time.* Evanston, IL: Northwestern University Press.

Gelman, S. A. (1999). The role of essentialism in children's concepts. In Reese, H. W. (Ed.), *Advances in child development and behavior, Vol. 27*. San Diego, CA: Academic Press.

Gergen, K., & Gergen, M. (1983). Narratives of the self. In Sarbin, T. R. & Schebe, K. E. (Eds.) *Studies in social identity*. New York: Praeger.

Gjerde, P. F., & Onishi, M. (2000). Selves, cultures, and nations: The psychological imagination of 'the Japanese' in the era of globalization. *Human Development*, **43**, 216–226.

Goldschmid-Bentler, M. L., & Bentler, P. M. (1968). The dimensions and measurement of conservation. *Child Development*, **39**(3), 787–802.

Grene, M. (1988). Hierarchies and behavior. In Greenberg, G. & Tobach, E. (Eds.), *Evolution of social behavior and integrative levels*. Hillsdale, NJ: Erlbaum.

Guardo, C. J., & Bohan, J. B. (1971). Development of a sense of self-identity in children. *Child Development*, **42**, 1909–1921.

Gutheil, G., & Rosengren, K. (1996). A rose by any other name: Preschoolers' understanding of individual identity across name and appearance changes. *British Journal of Developmental Psychology*, **14**(4), 477–498.

Habermas, J. (1985). Questions and counterquestions (J. Bohman, Trans.). In Bernstein, R. J. (Ed.), *Habermas and modernity*. Cambridge, MA: MIT Press.

Hacking, I. (1995). *Multiple personality and the science of memory?* Princeton, NJ: Princeton University Press.

Hacking, I. (1999). *The social construction of what?* Cambridge, MA: Harvard University Press.

Hall, D. G. (1998). Continuity and the persistence of objects: When the whole is greater than the sum of its parts. *Cognitive Psychology*, **37**, 28–59.

Harré, R. (1979). *Social being: A theory for social psychology*. Oxford: Blackwell.

Hart, D. J., Maloney, J., & Damon, W. (1987). The meaning and development of personal identity. In Honess, T. & Yardley, K. M. (Eds.) *Self and identity: Perspective across the lifespan*. London: Routledge & Kegan Paul.

Health Canada. (1991). *Statistical profile on native mental health (Background Report of the Statistical and Technical Working Group, Mental Health Advisory Services, Indian and Northern Health Services)*. Ottawa: Medical Services Branch Steering Committee on Native Mental Health, Medical Services Branch Health & Welfare Canada.

Hermans, H. J. (1996). Voicing the self: From information processing to dialogical interchange. *Psychological Bulletin*, **119**(1), 31–50.

Hermans, H. J. M., & Kempen, H. J. G. (1998). Moving cultures: The perilous problems of cultural dichotomies in a globalizing society. *American-Psychologist*, **53**(10), 1111–1120.

Hermans, H. J., Kempen, H. J., & Van Loon, R. J. (1992). The dialogical self: Beyond individualism and rationalism. *American Psychologist*, **47**(1), 23–33.

Hildebrand, D. K., Lange, J. D., & Rosenthal, H. (1977). *Prediction analysis of cross classifications*. New York: Wiley.

Hirsch, E. (1976). *The persistence of objects*. Philadelphia: University City Science Center.

Holden, C. (1986). Youth suicide: New research focuses on a growing social problem. *Science*, **233**, 839–841.

Holland, D. (1997). Selves as cultured. In Ashmore, R. & Jussin, L. (Eds.) *Self and identity: Fundamental issues*. New York: Oxford University Press.

Inagaki, K., & Sugiyama, K. (1988). Attributing human characteristics: Developmental changes in over- and underattribution. *Cognitive Development*, **3**, 55–70.

Ip, G. W. M., & Bond, M. H. (1995). Culture, values and the spontaneous self-concept. *Asian Journal of Psychology*, **1**, 29–35.

James, W. (1891). *The principles of psychology*. London: Macmillan.

James, W. (1910). *Psychology: The briefer course*. New York: Holt.

Kagitcibasi, C. (1996). *Family and human development across cultures: A view from the other side.* Mahwah, NJ: Erlbaum.

Keil, F. C. (1989). *Concepts, kinds, and cognitive development.* Cambridge, MA: MIT Press.

Kerby, A. P. (1991). *Narrative and the self.* Bloomington: Indiana University Press.

Kirmayer, L. (1994). Suicide among Canadian aboriginal people. *Transcultural Psychiatric Research Review,* **31,** 3–57.

Kitayama, S. (2002). Culture and basic psychological processes—Toward a system view of culture: Comment on Oyserman et al. (2002). *Psychological Bulletin,* **128**(1), 89–96.

Kitayama, S. & Markus, H. (Eds.). (1994). *Emotion and culture: Empirical studies of mutual influence.* Washington, DC: American Psychological Association.

Kontje, T. C. (1993). *The German Bildungsroman: History of a national genre.* Columbia, SC: Camden House.

Kuhn, M. H., & McPartland, T. S. (1954). An empirical investigation of self-attitudes. *American Sociological Review,* **19,** 68–76.

Lacan, J. (1968). *The language of the self, the function of language in psychoanalysis.* Baltimore: John Hopkins Press.

Lakoff, G., & Johnson, M. (1999). *Philosophy in the flesh: The embodied mind and its challenge to Western thought.* New York: Basic Books.

Lampinen, J. M., & Odegard, T. N., (2000, November). Diachronic disunity. University of Arkansas Symposium on Memory and the Self, Fayetteville, AR.

Lewis, M., & Ferrari, M. (2001). Cognitive-emotional self-organization in personality development and personal identity. In Bosma, H. A. & Kunnen, E. S. (Eds.) *Identity and emotions: A self-organizational perspective.* Cambridge, UK: Cambridge University Press.

Lightfoot, C. (1997). *The culture of adolescent risk-taking.* New York: Guilford Press.

Linehan, M., Goodstein, J., Nielsen, S., & Chiles, J. (1983). Reasons for staying alive when you are thinking of killing yourself: The reasons for living inventory. *Journal of Consulting and Clinical Psychology,* **51,** 276–286.

Locke, J. (1956). *Essay concerning human understanding.* Oxford: Clarendon Press. (Original work published 1694).

Lonner, W. J., & Adamopoulos, J. (1997). Culture as antecedent to behavior. In Berry, J. W. & Poortinga, Y. H. (Eds.) *Handbook of cross-cultural psychology. Vol. 1: Theory and method* (2nd ed). Needlam Heights, MA: Allyn and Bacon.

Luckman, T. (1979). Personal identity as an evolutionary and historical problem. In von Cranach, M. (Ed.), *Human ethology: Claims and limits of a new discipline.* New York: Cambridge University Press.

MacIntyre, A. (1977). Epistemological crisis, dramatic narrative, and the philosophy of science. *The Monist,* **60**(4), 453–472.

MacIntyre, A. (1984). *After virtue: A study in moral theory.* Notre Dame, IN: University of Notre Dame Press.

Mandler, J. M. (1984). *Stories, scripts, and scenes: Aspects of schema theory.* Hillsdale, NJ: Erlbaum.

Marcia, J. E. (1966). Development and validation of ego identity status. *Journal of Personality and Social Psychology,* **5,** 551–558.

Maris, R. (1981). *Pathways to suicide: A survey of self-destructive behaviors.* Baltimore: Johns Hopkins University.

Markus, H. R., & Kitayama, S. (1991). Culture and the self: Implications for cognition, emotion, and motivation. *Psychological Review,* **98,** 224–253.

Marr, D. (1982). *Vision: A computational investigation into the human representation and processing of visual information.* New York: W. H. Freeman.

REFERENCES

Matsumoto, C. (1999). Culture and self: An empirical assessment of Markus and Kitayama's theory of independent and interdependent self-construal. *Asian Journal of Social Psychology*, **2**, 289–310.

McAdams, D., Diamond, A., de, St.Aubin, & Mansfield, E. (1997). Stories of commitment: the psychosocial construction of generative lives. *Journal of Personality and Social Psychology*, **72**(3), 678–694.

McQuillan, M. (2000). *The narrative reader.* London: Routledge.

Medin, D. L. (1989). Concepts and conceptual structure. *American Psychologist*, **44**, 1469–1481.

Meehan, P., Lamb, J., & Saltzmen, L. (1992). Attempted suicide among young adults: Progress toward a meaningful estimate of prevalence. *American Journal of Psychiatry*, **149**, 41–44.

Melges, F., & Weisz, A. (1971). The personal future and suicidal ideation. *The Journal of Nervous and Mental Disease*, **153**, 244–250.

Miller, J. G. (1996). Theoretical issues in cultural psychology. In Berry, J. W. , Poortinga, Y. H. & Pandley, J. (Eds.) *Handbook of cross-cultural psychology. Vol. 1, Theory and method.* Boston: Allyn & Bacon.

Miller, J. G. (2002). Bringing culture to basic psychological theory—Beyond individualism and collectivism: Comment on Oyserman et al. (2002). *Psychological Bulletin*, **128**(1), 97–109.

Mink, L. O. (1969). History and fiction as modes of comprehension. *New Literary History*, **1**, 541–558.

Mishler, E. G. (1995). Models of narrative analysis: A typology. *Journal of Narrative and Life History*, **5**, 87–123.

Nannis, E. D., & Cowan, P. A. (Eds.), (1988). *Developmental psychopathology and its treatment.* San Francisco: Jossey-Bass.

Neuringer, C., & Harris, R. M. (1974). The perception of the passage of time among death-involved hospital patients. *Life-Threatening Behavior*, **2**, 240–254.

Noam, G. G., Chandler, M. J., & Lalonde, C. (1995). Clinical-developmental psychology: Constructivism and social cognition in the study of psychological dysfunctions. In Cicchetti, D. & Cohen, D. (Eds.) *Handbook of developmental psychopathology, Vol. 1.* New York: Wiley.

Norenzayan, A., Choi, I., & Nisbett, R. E. (1999). Eastern and Western perceptions of causality for social behavior: Lay theories about personalities and situations. In Prentice, D. A. & Miller, D. T. (Eds.) *Cultural divides: Understanding and overcoming group conflict.* New York: Russell Sage.

Overton, W. F. (1998). Developmental psychology: Philosophy, concepts, and methodology. In Damon, W. (Series Ed.) Lerner, R. M. (Vol. Ed.), *The handbook of child psychology. Vol. 1, Theoretical models of human development* (5th ed). New York: Wiley.

Oyserman, D., Coon, H., & Kemmelmeier, M. (2002). Rethinking individualism and collectivism: Evaluation of theoretical assumptions and meta-analyses. *Psychological Bulletin*, **128**(1), 3–72.

Parfit, D. (1971). Personal identity. *Philosophical Review*, **80**(1), 3–27.

Peevers, B. H. (1987). The self as observer of the self: A developmental analysis of the subjective self. In Howes, T. & Yardley, K. M. (Eds.), *Self and identity: Perspective across the lifespan* (pp. 147–158). London: Routledge & Kegan Paul.

Pennebaker, J. W., & Graybeal, A. (2001). Patterns of natural language use: Disclosure, personality, and social integration. *Current Directions in Psychological Science*, **10**, 90–93.

Pennebaker, J. W., & King, L. A. (1999). Linguistic styles: Language use as an individual difference. *Journal of Personality and Social Psychology*, **77**(6), 1296–1312.

Pennebaker, J. W., & Lay, T. C., (2002). Language use and personality during crises: Analyses of Mayor. Rudolph Guiliani's press conference. *Journal of Research in Personality*, **36**, 27–282.

Pennebaker, J. W., & Stone, L. D. (in press). Words of wisdom: Language use over the lifespan. *Journal of Personality*.

Perry, J. (1976). The importance of being identical. In Rorty, A. O. (Ed.), *The identities of persons*. Berkeley: University of California Press.

Pfeffer, C. R. (1986). *The suicidal child*. New York: Guilford Press.

Phinney, J. (1992). The Multigroup Ethnic Identity Measure: A new scale for use with adolescents and young adults from diverse groups. *Journal of Adolescent Research*, **7**, 156–176.

Piaget, J. (1968). *On the development of of memory and identity* (E. Duckworth, Trans.) Barre, MA: Clark University Press/Barre Publishers.

Piaget, J. (1970). Piaget's theory. In Mussen, P. (Ed.), *Carmichael's manual of child psychology*, Vol. 1. New York: Wiley.

Polkinghorne, C. (1988). *Narrative knowing and the human sciences*. Albany, NY: SUNY Press.

Putnam, H. (1988). *Representation and reality*. Cambridge, MA: MIT Press.

Report of the Royal Commission on Aboriginal Peoples. (1996). Hull, Quebec: Canada Communications Group Publishing.

Resnik, H. L., & Dizmang, L. H. (1971). Observations on suicidal behavior among American Indians. *American Journal of Psychiatry*, **127**(7), 882–887.

Ricoeur, P. (1983). Can fiction narratives be true? *Analecta Husserliana*, **14**, 3–19.

Ricoeur, P. (1985). History as narrative and practice. *Philosophy Today*, **29**, 213–222.

Riessman, C. K. (1993). *Narrative analysis*. Newbury Park, CA: Sage Publications.

Ring, M. (1987). *Beginning with the pre-Socratics*. Mountain View, CA: Mayfield.

Rodin, J. (1986). Aging and health: Effects of the sense of control. *Science*, **233**, 1271–1276.

Rogers, L., & Kegan, R. (1990). Mental growth and mental health as distinct concepts in the study of developmental psychopathology: Theory, research, and clinical implications. In Keating, D. & Rosen, H. (Eds.) *Constructivist perspectives on developmental psychopathology and atypical development*. Hillsdale, NJ: Erlbaum.

Rorty, A. O. (1973). The transformations of persons. *Philosophy*, **48**, 261–275.

Rorty, A. O. (1976). *The identities of persons*. Berkeley: University of California Press.

Rorty, A. O. (1987). Persons as rhetorical categories. *Social Research*, **54**(1), 55–72.

Rosengren, K. S., Gelman, S. A, Kalish, C. W., & McCormick, M. (1991). As time goes by: Children's early understanding of growth in animals. *Child Development*, **62**(6), 1302–1320.

Ross, C. P. (1985). Teaching children facts of life and death: Suicide prevention in the schools. In Peck, M. L. , Farberow, N. L. & Litman, R. E. (Eds.) *Youth suicide*. New York: Springer.

Rubenstein, J. L., Heeren, T., Housman, D., Rubin, C., & Stechler, G. (1988, March). Suicidal behaviour in "normal" adolescents: Risk and protective factors. Paper presented at the Biennial Meeting of the Society for Research in Adolescence, Alexandria, VA.

Ryder, A. G., Alden, L. E., & Paulus, D. L. (2000). Is acculturation unidimensional or bidimensional? A head-to-head comparison in the prediction of personality, self-identity, and adjustment. *Journal of Personality and Social Psychology*, **79**(1), 49–65.

Schlesinger, A. (1977). The modern consciousness and the winged chariot. In Gorman, B. & Wessman, A. (Eds.) *The personal experience of time*. New York: Plenum.

Schneidman, E. S. (1985). *Definition of suicide*. New York: Wiley.

Shaffer, D. (1985). Depression, mania, and suicidal acts. In Rutter, M. & Hersov, L. (Eds.) *Child and adolescent psychiatry: Modern approaches*. New York: Guilford Press.

Shalom, A. (1985). *The body-mind conceptual framework and the problem of personal identity.* Atlantic Highlands, NJ: Humanities Press International.

Shotter, J. (1984). *Social accountability and selfhood.* Oxford: Basil Blackwell.

Singelis, T. M. (1994). The measurement of independent and interdependent self-construals. *Personality and Social Psychology Bulletin,* **20**, 580–591.

Smith, P. (1988). *Discerning the subject.* Minneapolis: University of Minnesota Press.

Smye, L. S. (1990). Control and health: An epidemiological perspective. In Rodin, J., Schooler, C. & Schaie, K. W. (Eds.), *Self-directedness: Causes and effects during the life course.* Hilldsdale, NJ: Erlbaum.

Spence, D. (1982). *Narrative truth and historical truth: Meaning and interpretation in psychoanalysis.* New York: Norton.

Strawson, G. (1999). Self and body: Self, body, and experience. *Supplement to the Proceedings of the Aristotelian-Society,* **73**, 307–332.

Szapocznik, J., Scopetta, M. A., Kurtines, W., & Aranalde, M. D. (1978). Theory and measurement of acculturation. *Revista Interamericana de Psicologia,* **12**(2), 113–130.

Taylor, C. (1988). The moral topography of the self. In *Hermeneutics and Psychological Theory.* New Brunswick, NJ: Princeton University Press.

Taylor, C. (1991). *The malaise of modernity.* Concord, Ontario: House of Anansi Press.

Triandis, H. (1989). The self and social behavior in differing cultural contexts. *Psychological Review,* **96**, 506–520.

Tulving, E. (1983). *Elements of episodic memory.* New York: Oxford University Press.

Turiel, E. (2002). *The culture of morality: Social development, context, and conflict.* Cambridge: Cambridge University Press.

Turiel, E., & Wainryb, C. (1994). Social reasoning and the varieties of social experiences in cultural contexts. In Reese, H. W. (Ed.), *Advances in child development and behavior* (**Vol 25.**). New York: Academy Press.

Turner, M. (1996). *The literary mind.* New York: Oxford University Press.

Tylor, E. B. (1874). *Primitive culture: Researches into the development of mythology, philosophy, religion, language, art, and custom.* London: J. Murray.

Unger, R. (1975). *Knowledge and politics.* New York: Free Press.

Updike, J. (1989). *Self consciousness: Memoirs.* New York: Knopf.

van Inwagen, P. (1990). Four-dimensional objects. *Nous,* **24**, 245–255.

Verkuyten, M. (1989). Self-concept in cross-cultural perspective: Turkish and Dutch adolescents in the Netherlands. *Journal of Social Psychology,* **129**, 184–185.

von Eye, A. (1997). Prediction Analysis Program for 32 bit Operation Systems. *Methods of Psychological Research Online,* **2**(2). (Internet: http://www.pabst-publishers.de/mpr/).

von Eye, A., & Brandtstädter, J. (1988). Evaluating developmental hypotheses using statement calculus and nonparametric statistics. In Baltes, P. & Lerner, R. (Eds.), *Life-span development and behavior: Vol. 8.* Hillsdale, NJ: Erlbaum.

Ward, C., & Rana-Deuba, A. (1999). Acculturation and adaptation revisited. *Journal of Cross-Cultural Psychology,* **30**, 373–392.

Watkins, D., Adair, J., Akande, A., Gerong, A., McInerney, D., Sunar, D., Watson, S., Wen, Q. F., & Wondimu, H. (1998). Individualism-collectivism, gender and the self-concept: A nine culture investigation. *Psychologia,* **41**, 259–271.

Watkins, D., & Regmi, M. (1996). Within-culture and gender differences in self-concept. An investigation with rural and urban Nepalese school children. *Journal of Cross-Cultural Psychology,* **27**, 692–699.

Watkins, D., Yau, J., Dahlin, B., & Wondimu, H. (1997). The Twenty Statements Test: Some measurement issues. *Journal of Cross-Cultural Psychology,* **28**, 626–633.

Weintraub, K. J. (1975). Autobiography and historical consciousness. *Critical Inquiry*, June, 821–848.
Wellman, H. (1990). *The child's theory of mind*. Cambridge, MA: MIT Press.
Wells, L. E., & Marwell, G. (1976). *Self-esteem: Its conceptualization and measurement*. London: Sage.
Whittaker, E. (1992). The birth of the anthropological self and its career. *Ethos*, **20**, 191–219.
Wiggins, D. (1980). *Sameness and substance*. Cambridge, MA: Harvard University Press.
Wildgen, W. (1994). *Process, image, and meaning: A realistic model of the meaning of sentences and narrative texts*. Philadelphia: John Benjamins.
Yufit, R. I., & Benzies, B. (1973). Assessing suicidal potential by time perspective. *Life-Threatening Behavior*, **3**, 270–282.
Zagorin, P. (1999). History, the referent, and narrative: Reflections on postmodernism now. *History and Theory*, **38**, 1–24.
Zygmuntowiscz, C. E., Burack, J. A., Evans, D. W., Klaiman, C., Mandour, T., Randolph, B., & Iarocci, G. (2000, June). *Cultural identity as a protective factor: A study of depression and problem behaviors in First Nations adolescents from an isolated community*. Poster presented at the annual meeting of the Jean Piaget Society, Montréal, Canada.

ACKNOWLEDGEMENTS

The list of persons and organizations that facilitated the work reported here, and to whom we are deeply indebted, is long and roughly divides itself into five categories. First, there are those who labored to help gather and organize the data that we report. In this group we wish to express our thanks to our immediate working colleagues Ulrich Teucher and Jesse Phillips of University of British Columbia's Department of Psychology; to Samaya Jardey and Florence Williams of the Squamish First Nation and Marla Jack and Caroline Frank of the Ahousaht First Nation; to Julie Cruikshank, Lisa Maberly, Holly Pommier, Michelle Morgan, and David Paul of the University of British Columbia; to Aislin Martin and Catherine Horvath of the University of Victoria; and to Grace Iarocci and Christopher Jones of Simon Fraser University. We also wish to acknowledge the special contributions of Lorraine Ball and of Michael Boyes to the earliest stages of this work.

A second category includes those persons and organizations who were particularly helpful in providing access to young persons and to databases that were critical to the completion of this project. We are particularly indebted to both the Squamish and Ahousaht First Nations for granting us permission to work within their traditional territories to gather the data reported in Study Five, to utilize their facilities, and for the privilege of working in partnership with members of their band and tribal councils. We are especially grateful for the assistance of Marlene Atleo, Pam Jack, and Louis Joseph of the Ahousaht Holistic Centre, the band councils of the Ahousaht and Squamish First Nations, and chiefs Bill Williams (Squamish) and Richard Atleo (Ahousaht). We are also appreciative of the cooperation offered by the teachers and administrators of the Richmond Christian High School. The staffs at Indian and Northern Affairs Canada and within the Office of the Chief Coroner of British Columbia and the Provincial Health Officer of British Columbia provided invaluable aid in our efforts to assemble the epidemiological suicide data set.

Group three in this list includes funding agencies: the Social Sciences and Humanities Research Council of Canada, the Universities of British Columbia and Victoria, The Human Early Learning Partnership, the Canadian Institutes for Health Research, and the Michael Smith Foundation for Health Research.

Fourth, we owe our most sincere thanks to the young men and women of Ahousaht, Squamish, and Richmond who volunteered their time and energy to participate in this research.

Fifth, and finally, we want to express our special appreciation to our three anonymous reviews, and especially to our editor Willis Overton, whose wise council and generous advice contributed in indispensable ways to the shaping and quality of this *Monograph*.

For correspondence, contact Michael J. Chandler, Department of Psychology, University of British Columbia, 2136 West Mall, Vancouver, British Columbia V6T 1Z4, Canada (chandler@interchange.ubc.ca).

COMMENTARY

TREADING FEARLESSLY: A COMMENTARY ON PERSONAL PERSISTENCE, IDENTITY DEVELOPMENT, AND SUICIDE

James E. Marcia

I found myself trying to answer the question the authors of this *Monograph* pose: How would I account for my own personal persistence in the face of the knowledge that I am physically and experientially a different person from whom I was yesterday and all the days before? Looking at pictures of a little boy in a play Marine outfit standing beside his uncle in a World War II Army uniform, I ask: How do I know that that little boy is (was) me? Similarly, looking at a string of other photos at different ages, I could pictorially trace the changes that have brought "me" to the current point of being. I am no longer those presentations of me, but I am still me. My introspective answer to this initial question is: memory and representation.

The internal and enduring me rests on remembered events in my life, on which I rely for a sense of continuity, like pearls strung along a temporal memory strand. If that strand of memories, and the meanings I give them, were severed by some kind of amnesia, my sense of personal continuity would vanish. However, what would likely not vanish would be my need to *construct* some such memory string. I would search, probably frantically, for items (drivers' license, passport, etc.) that would allow me to re-construct and confirm my identity in the world. But even these gathered events would need to make an inner resonant connection.

What is especially interesting to me is that most persons seem to have a need to do this—to construct and maintain some sense of continuity. It is adaptive to do so. If I could not bundle up pertinent parts of my previous life events and experience them as "mine," I would not be able to anticipate the future and I would have to face every situation as if it were brand new.

Unless I had very attentive caretakers, I would not survive one street crossing. It seems to me, then, that the basis for self-continuity lies in memory, just as the basis for an eventual identity lies in a secure sense of self.

Many of my following comments will have to do more with additional thoughts and questions regarding material the authors have presented than with criticism of their work. I have already spoken of "memory" and I shall later speak of "pain." What the authors are looking at—self-persistence, identity, and suicide—relates to memory, a faculty that goes to the heart of what it means to be human. We could truly be called "the remembering animal." And whether our memories are veridical or constructed (or both, which is most likely), they furnish us with our sense of a continuing self. This sense of a continuing self is a necessary, but not a sufficient, condition for an identity. Memory and the ensuing self tell us *that* we are. Identity, as I understand it, is a later developmental attainment that tells us *what* and *who* we are.

The research that my colleagues and I have done on identity springs from an origin different from that of authors' research presented in this *Monograph*. Our studies on identity status (Marcia, Waterman, Matteson, Archer, & Orlofsky, 1993) began as an attempt to validate Erik Erikson's (1980) ego psychoanalytic theory of psychosocial development. We initially were interested in how late adolescents go about managing the transition from adolescence to adulthood in terms of shifts in occupational and ideological perspectives and the eventual formation of an ego identity. Subsequently, our interests have focused on how adults maintain or shift their ego identity (see Marcia, 2002; Strayer, 2002). The authors of the present *Monograph* began their work from the philosophical perspective of a theory of mind within a general Piagetian orientation. They are interested in how one explains one's own and others' continuity in light of obvious and inevitable physical and psychological discontinuities. These two approaches coincide and complement each other in at least two ways. They both focus on the developmental period of adolescence, when discontinuity becomes especially acute, and they both assume the formation of psychological structures over time. Furthermore, both agree that adolescents cannot remain who they were as children or they will fare poorly in an adult world. Yet, they must retain some sense of continuity or they risk alienation from their past and perhaps that sense of anomie that Durkheim related to suicide.

The relationships between cognitive development (à la Piaget) and identity development (à la Erikson) have been investigated previously. Some of this work is summarized in Marcia et al., 1993; Marcia, 1994; and Marcia,1999. In general, the relation of identity to such variables as formal operational thought, levels of moral reasoning (Kohlberg & Kramer, 1969), stages of epistemic thought (Boyes & Chandler, 1992; Peterson, Marcia, &

Carpendale, in press), and cognitive sophistication (MacKinnon & Marcia, 2002) have been correlational in nature. Advanced identity formation is associated with advanced reasoning ability. It seems that adolescents and adults who can take multiple perspectives on themselves and others also have a firmer and more flexible sense of who they are. Although they are not necessarily happier for it (see Hearn et al., under review), they seem not to experience the levels of despair found in less cognitively sophisticated persons (Noam, Chandler, & Lalonde, 1995, cited in the present *Monograph*). This relation between cognition and affect needs further discussion.

The authors are particularly persuasive in the first sections of the *Monograph* where they present their empirically buttressed argument that lack of self-continuity warranting is associated with increased suicide risk. They demonstrate that among hospitalized youth, those having no self-continuity warranting strategy are higher in suicide risk than those having some warranting strategy. The question I have concerns *why* the self-warranting process becomes derailed. It might be a combination of psychological pain, especially acute during adolescent transitional points, coupled with increased formal operational capabilities that lead the adolescent to question previous warranting strategies. Bereft of previous cognitive safeguards that permit one to say "Things are bad, but they've been bad before and I've survived," pain seems to be all that exists and death today is preferable to waking up in the same condition tomorrow. Pain has become synonymous with self and any conception of past and future is foreshortened to the immediate excruciating present.

The engagement of self-warranting strategies requires maintaining perspective, and that is just what psychological pain obliterates. The hospitalized may not have killed themselves because they have some remnant of hope remaining, because they do not have enough energy available to act, or, most likely, because they are in the care of others who *do* have the sense of perspective necessary to possess such self-warranting strategies—both for themselves and those in their care. The foregoing is not so different from what the authors have said, except that it places pain (affect) rather than thought (cognition) in the foreground (see also Strayer, 2002). This is important in terms of intervention. I don't believe, and I don't believe that the authors believe, that teaching self-warranting strategies would be an effective technique in forestalling adolescent suicide. We would probably agree that buying some time in the form of providing a protective setting would be a first therapeutic step, followed by hours of listening that would allow for the likely naturally occurring self-continuity warranting process to be reestablished.

It should be noted that it is only *levels* of warranting, not the warranting strategies themselves (i.e., Narrative and Essentialist), that demonstrate a relation to suicidality. Further, these levels of warranting (within the Essentialist track) were found in a prior investigation to be highly related to a measure of Piagetian cognitive competence. This measure, assessed via the Goldschmid-Bentler Conservation Assessment Task, was dropped after its demonstrated usefulness as a validating variable. Would the cognitive competence measure also have predicted suicidality? If it did, that might suggest that suicidal youths have a general cognitive derailment that underlies more specific difficulties in self-warranting.

From a comparison of the warranting strategies of hospitalized suicidal adolescents and "normal" youths, the authors of this *Monograph* move to the social issue of cultural continuity and aboriginal youth suicide. The authors might have begun this task by undertaking construct validation for their newly formulated warranting tracks, Essentialist and Narrative, and the levels of warranting within these strategies. To this point in the *Monograph* they had established only that these strategies can be reliably discriminated and scored. However, rather than pursuing the path of further construct validation, they move to tackle a social issue with their newly minted constructs. Why make this leap if the appropriate next step might be to demonstrate that the Essentialist and Narrative strategies relate in expected ways to other similar measures (concurrent validity) and to show that they have a predictable impact on theoretically expectable outcomes (predictive validity)?

I think that the new constructs proposed in this work were pressed into service because these researchers, like all of us, live in a particular context (which I happen to share) with its pressing contextual demands. It is impossible to be a social scientist in British Columbia and not be aware of the high incidence of Native youth suicide. Perhaps the investigatory leap taken by the authors is justified given the potential societal impact and the urgent need to address the high suicide rate among Aboriginal youth. Nevertheless, much more work needs to be undertaken within mainstream communities on these new concepts and their implications for normal adolescent development. That this can be done is shown by the efforts of applied developmentalists such as Irving Sigel who used his Piagetian-based research on "distancing strategies" to help initiate and guide Project Head Start in largely urban Black communities in the United States in the 1960s and 1970s.

The authors make a case for a similarity between individual self-continuity and cultural self-continuity. Although this is conceptually appealing, and to some extent convincing, we again come up against the issues of construct validity. The only empirical evidence of some validity for the "cultural continuity" construct lies in the lower youth suicide rates for bands higher in this variable, and that finding does not bear directly on the construct itself. Moreover, labels other than "culturally continuous" might be given to bands showing lower suicide rates. They might be called "successful negotiators," "high self-esteem," etc. If the latter were the best characterization, then one could write a different story: Youth growing up in bands that have come to esteem themselves highly, as evidenced by such actions as their persistence at successful negotiations with the government, insistence on provision of adequate social services, and establishment of self-governance, provide a more self-enhancing context within which their adolescents grow up.

Further, if adolescents in this context had higher levels of self-warranting, would this be the primary causative factor in lower suicidality or a by-product of other factors such as self-esteem, more youth activities, hope for a satisfactory economic future with a variety of viable occupational niches, etc? The problem lies with the establishment of construct validity for "cultural continuity." What are its other predictive implications and what is the relation between these and individual levels of self-continuity warranting, and what is path leading from cultural discontinuity to higher youth suicide rates? Without this information, we are left with a tantalizing and plausible, but not demonstrated, possibility of a connection between cultural continuity, Native youth warranting levels, and suicide. In the series of studies presented in this *Monograph* the relations between cultural continuity and warranting tracks or levels remain undemonstrated. I, however, remain optimistic that such a demonstration will be forthcoming.

In the last study reported in the *Monograph*, the authors do a superb job of establishing reliability, both interscorer and test-retest, for their measure. In addition, they examine story stimulus content differences and presentation medium differences. They also establish some discriminant validity for their warranting measure by looking at its relation to indices of linguistic sophistication, self-understanding, idiocentrism/allocentrism, and ethnic identification. This section is an almost ideal model of measure construction. Some concurrent validity is furnished by the finding that Essentialists have a more "static entity" orientation in their implicit personality theory preferences, whereas Narrativists have a more "process" orientation. Predictive validity, however, is scarce except for the fact that the measure establishes differences between Native and non-Native warranting styles. No rationale is given for *why* these two groups should differ, or even, after the fact, why they did differ. But that the authors have a strong measure with which to do further research and that the two groups, at least as constituted in this study, do differ is unquestionable. Clearly, further work needs to be done on establishing a more substantial nomological network for the constructs of Essentialism and Narrativity as well as "cultural continuity."

I think that what the authors want to be able to say is that both Level of self-warranting and Track of self-warranting are related to suicidality in

Native youth. The narrative might go like this. The lower the Level of self-warranting, the greater the risk of suicide in adolescents in general. Individuals, such as Native youth, who employ Narrative strategies may be more dependent on context than are Essentialist youth. Hence, they might be especially vulnerable to cultural discontinuity (i.e., sink to lower warranting levels). Following from this, the risk of Native adolescent suicidality could be lowered if cultural continuity in Native communities were supported and maintained. Essentialist warranting strategies might be less vulnerable to cultural factors. If one has become convinced that one has some kind of inner core, unassailable by cultural vicissitudes, then one's self-warranting might be less vulnerable to external factors. However, this would be only a matter of degree. We don't know how many of those suicidal hospitalized youth used an Essentialist or Narrative strategy, but we can assume that some, if not most, of them had been employing an Essentialist track. It might be the case that Essentialists' strength is more "brittle" and that once shattered is less amenable to repair by positive cultural factors. Hence, while Narrativists may be more susceptible to cultural discontinuities, Essentialists, once breached, may be less amenable to cultural support. Demonstration of this possibility seems, empirically, a long way off.

If the authors don't want to say that there is a relationship between Tracks and Levels of warranting in suicidality among Native youth, in particular, then it is difficult to see why these variables are all included in one monograph. There is no evidence presented that either Narrative strategies or level of warranting are especially vulnerable to cultural discontinuity. Nor is there any established relation between Narrativity at low levels and suicidality. The only suicidality data (from the hospitalized, non-Native sample) concern Level, not Track × Level. Although these can be woven together rhetorically, the empirical evidence is lacking. More work needs to be done before such promising ideas can be confirmed. What we do know for certain is that the authors have developed and begun to validate what promises to be a very good five-level measure of Essentialism/Narrativity. They are certainly well-poised to establish the missing links. One of the criteria for the publication of a work as an *SRCD Monograph* is that it "should start a new field or put an end to an old one." The present *Monograph* clearly begins, but does not end, an exciting and promising field of inquiry.

There is no question that a sense of continuity is an essential aspect of identity viewed from a developmental perspective, whether one starts from the basis of a theory of mind or an ego psychoanalytic theory. The ego psychoanalytic approach furnishes a broader life-span perspective in that it views identity as developing throughout the life cycle and places adolescence within a lifetime developmental context. However, breadth has its downside: a risk of superficiality and nonspecificity. The work presented here furnishes a more fine-grained approach to the continuity aspect of identity than has been found in the identity status research. Yet, an interesting connection might be made between the work of these researchers and that of Michael Berzonsky (1989), who investigated extensively the information-processing styles of the identity statuses. He described an "informational" style (an openness to identity disconfirming data) as characterizing Identity Achievement persons, those who have gone through a decision-making process and made commitments in important life areas. A "normative" style (information selectively filtered to confirm an existing identity) is typical of Foreclosure individuals, those who are committed but have done little exploring. A "diffuse" style (a scattered, unfocused approach) is related to Identity Diffusionists who are uncommitted and who have undergone little genuine exploration.

It is the focus on *process* that ties these two bodies of work together. Berzonsky discussed different ways in which adolescents deal with identity-relevant information; Chandler and his colleagues are more concerned with underlying cognitive developmental structures that might enable those processing styles. One could imagine coordinating three lines of work. Individuals with the lowest levels of self-persistence warranting would likely be "diffuse" in their information-processing style and be categorized as Identity Diffusionists on an identity status interview. They, together with persons in the Moratorium status, those who are moving out of a Foreclosed position into an "identity crisis," would likely be at the highest suicidal risk. Individuals at moderate levels of self-warranting who employ a "normative" style would likely be Foreclosures, those "brittle" Essentialists mentioned previously. These persons suffer from too much self-persistence; they are who they've always been—with a vengeance. Finally, individuals who are at more sophisticated levels of self-warranting and who pursue an "information"-oriented processing strategy would likely be Identity Achievers and the most resistant to suicidality. If one looked back developmentally to eras prior to adolescence, one would likely find the same intertwined strands of cognitive development and psychosocial development that we have found in our identity status research. And if one were to prescribe familial and cultural conditions to enhance both cognitive and psychosocial development, these conditions would likely be identical (see Marcia, 1999).

When we look to the larger picture, we note that Erik Erikson furnished us with a general outline of what we might expect in terms of psychosocial development at adolescence. However, he was not at all specific about the developmental processes occurring within that stage. If we expect to be able to intervene effectively, whether on an individual or social basis, we must know about these underlying processes, both what enhances them and what derails them. Identity status research has provided the variables of exploration and commitment in important life areas. Berzonsky's "identity style" approach has suggested differing information-processing modes characteristic of the identity statuses. And the work presented here by Chandler and his colleagues, in addition to providing another potential liaison between Erikson and Piaget, furnishes an empirically based strategy for investigating an essential aspect of adolescent identity: the maintenance of a sense of personal persistence or self-continuity. More than the other two approaches, the present researchers have carried their investigations into some of the darkest and most difficult problem areas of the real world. Even though some empirical links may be missing, this is important and potentially life-saving research. Not many of us can say that about our work.

References

Berzonsky, M. D. (1989). Identity style: Conceptualization and measurement. *Journal of Adolescent Research*, **4**, 267–281.

Boyes, M., & Chandler, M. J. (1992). Cognitive development, epistemic doubt, and identity formation in adolescence. *Journal of Youth and Adolescence*, **21**(3), 277–304.

Durkheim, E. (1951). *Suicide: A Study in Sociology*. Toronto: Collier-McMillan. (original work published 1897)

Erikson, E. H. (1980). *Identity and the life cycle: A re-issue*. New York: Norton.

Hearn, S., Saulnier, G., Strayer, J., Glenham, M., Koopman, R., & Marcia, J. E. (under review). Between integrity and despair: Toward construct validation of Erikson's eighth stage. Department of Psychology, Simon Fraser University, Burnaby, British Columbia, Canada.

Kohlberg, L., & Kramer, R. (1969). Continuities and discontinuities in childhood and adult moral development. *Human Development*, **12**, 93–120.

MacKinnon, J., & Marcia, J. E. (2002). Concurring patterns of women's identity status, attachment styles, and understanding of children's development. *International Journal of Behavioral Development*, **26**(1), 70–81.

Marcia, J. E. (1994). Ego identity and object relations. In Masling, J. & Bornstein, R. F. (Eds.) *Empirical perspectives on object relations theory* (pp. 59–103). Washington, D.C.: American Psychological Association.

Marcia, J. E. (1999). Representational thought in ego identity, psychotherapy, and psychosocial developmental theory. In Sigel, I. E. (Ed.) *Development of mental representation: Theories and applications* (pp. 391–414). Mahwah, NJ: Erlbaum.

Marcia, J. E. (2002). Identity and psychosocial development in adulthood. *Identity: An International Journal of Theory and Research*, **2**(1), 7–29.

Marcia, J. E., Waterman, A. S., Matteson, D. R., Archer, S. L., & Orlofsky, J. I. (1993). *Ego identity: A handbook for psychosocial research*. New York: Springer-Verlag.

Noam, G. G., Chandler, J. J., & Lalonde, C. E. (1995). Clinical-developmental psychology: Constructivism and social cognition in the study of psychological dysfunctions. In Cicchetti, D. & Cohen, D. (Eds.) *Handbook of Developmental Psychopathology: Volume I* (pp. 424–466). New York: Wiley.

Peterson, D. M., Marcia, J. E., & Carpendale, J. (in press). Identity: Does thinking make it so?

Sigel, I. E. (1970). The distancing hypothesis: A causal hypothesis for the acquisition of representational thought. In M. Jones (Ed.), *The effects of early experience*. Miami, FL: University of Miami.

Strayer, J. (2002). The dynamics of emotion and life cycle identity. *Identity: An International Journal of Theory and Research*, **2**(1), 47–79.

CONTRIBUTORS

Michael J. Chandler is Distinguished CIHR/MSFHR Professor in Developmental Psychology at the University of British Columbia in Vancouver, Canada. His research centers on the study of young people's social-cognitive development, especially as such age-related changes bear on matters of interest to developmental psychopathologists and health professionals. Most recently his work has come to focus on cross-cultural comparisons of epistemic and identity development as these differently unfold in Canada's Aboriginal and culturally mainstream youth.

Christopher E. Lalonde is an assistant professor in the Department of Psychology at the University of Victoria. His research interests include social-cognitive development in childhood and adolescence and the influence of culture on identity development and determinants of health.

Bryan W. Sokol is an assistant professor in the Department of Psychology at Simon Fraser University. In addition to his interests in identity development, Bryan's research includes the study of children's developing epistemic and moral reasoning.

Darcy Hallett is a Ph.D. candidate in Developmental Psychology at the University of British Columbia. In addition to the subject matter of this *Monograph* and to identity development in general, Darcy's research interests include epistemological development and children's understanding of mathematics.

James Marcia is currently Professor Emeritus Simon Fraser University and formerly Professor of Clinical/Developmental Psychology and Director of the Psychological Clinic at Simon Fraser. His research interests involve the construct validation of psychosocial developmental theory, and the development of identity.

STATEMENT OF EDITORIAL POLICY

The *Monographs* series is devoted to publishing developmental research that generates authoritative new findings and uses these to foster fresh, better integrated, or more coherent perspectives on major developmental issues, problems, and controversies. The significance of the work in extending developmental theory and contributing definitive empirical information in support of a major conceptual advance is the most critical editorial consideration. Along with advancing knowledge on specialized topics, the series aims to enhance cross-fertilization among developmental disciplines and developmental sub fields. Therefore, clarity of the links between the specific issues under study and questions relating to general developmental processes is important. These links, as well as the manuscript as a whole, must be as clear to the general reader as to the specialist. The selection of manuscripts for editorial consideration, and the shaping of manuscripts through reviews-and-revisions, are processes dedicated to actualizing these ideals as closely as possible.

Typically *Monographs* entail programmatic large-scale investigations; sets of programmatic interlocking studies; or—in some cases—smaller studies with highly definitive and theoretically significant empirical findings. Multi-authored sets of studies that center on the same underlying question can also be appropriate; a critical requirement here is that all studies address common issues, and that the contribution arising from the set as a whole be unique, substantial, and well integrated. The needs of integration preclude having individual chapters identified by individual authors. In general, irrespective of how it may be framed, any work that is judged to significantly extend developmental thinking will be taken under editorial consideration.

To be considered, submissions should meet the editorial goals of *Monographs* and should be no briefer than a minimum of 80 pages (including references and tables). There is an upper limit of 175–200 pages. In exceptional circumstances this upper limit may be modified. (please submit four copies). Because a *Monograph* is inevitable lengthy and usually substantively complex, it is particularly important that the text be well organized and written in clear, precise, and literate English. Note, however, that authors from non-English-speaking countries should not be put off by this stricture. In accordance with the general aims of SRCD, this series is actively interested in promoting international exchange of developmental research. Neither membership in the Society nor affiliation with the academic discipline of psychology are relevant in considering a *Monographs* submission.

The corresponding author for any manuscript must, in the submission letter, warrant that all coauthors are in agreement with the content of the manuscript. The corresponding author also is responsible for informing all coauthors, in a timely manner, of manuscript submission, editorial decisions, reviews received, and any revisions recommended. Before publication, the corresponding author also must warrant in the submission letter that the study has been conducted according to the ethical guidelines of the Society for Research in Child Development.

Potential authors who may be unsure whether the manuscript they are planning would make an appropriate submission are invited to draft an outline of what they propose, and send it to the Editor for assessment. This mechanism, as well as a more detailed description of all editorial policies, evaluation process, and format requirements can be found at the Editorial Office web site (http://astro.temple.edu/-overton/monosrcd.html) or by contacting the Editor, Wills F. Overton, Temple University-Psychology, 1701 North 13th St. – Rm 567, Philadelphia, PA 19122-6085 (e-mail: monosrcd@temple.edu) (telephone: 1-215-204-7360).

Monographs of the Society for Reasearch in Child Development (ISSN 0037-976X), one of three publications of Society of Research in Child Development, is published three times a year by Blackwell Publishing, Inc., with offices at 350 Main Street, Malden, MA 02148, USA, and 9600 Garsington Road, Oxford OX4 2DQ, UK. Call 800-835-6770 or 781-388-8200 (US office) or +44-1865-251866 (UK office) or Fax: 781-388-8232 or +44-1865-381393. e-mail: subscrip@blackwellpublishing.com, on the web www.blackwellpublishing.com/cservices. A subscription to *Monographs of the SRCD* comes with a subscription to *Child Development* (published six times a year in February, April, June, August, October and December).

INFORMATION FOR SUBSCRIBERS For new orders, renewals, sample copy requests, claims, change of address, and all other subscription correspondence, please contact the Journals Subscription Department at the publisher's Malden Office.

INSTITUTIONAL PREMIUM RATES* FOR MONOGRAPHS OF THE SRCD /CHILD DEVELOPMENT 2003 The Americas $375, Rest of World £268. Customers in Canada should add 7% CST to The Americas price or provide evidence of entitlement to exemption. Customers in the UK and EU should add VAT at 5% or provide a VAT registration number or evidence of entitlement to exemption.

*Includes print plus premium online access to the current and all available backfiles. Print and online-only rates are also available. For more information about Blackwell Publishing journals, including online access information, terms and conditions, and other pricing options, please visit www.blackwellpublishing.com or contact our customer service department, tel: 1 800 835-6770 or +1 781 388-8206 (US office); +44 (0)1865 251866 (UK office).

INSTITUTIONAL SUBSCRIPTION RATES FOR MONOGRAPHS OF THE SRCD/ CHILD DEVELOPMENT/CHILD DEVELOPMENT ABSTRACTS AND BIBLIOGRA-PHY 2002 The Americas $369, Rest of World £246. All orders must be paid by credit card, business check, or money order. Checks and money orders should be made payable to Blackwell Publishers. Canadian residents please add 7% GST. V.

BACK ISSUES Back issues are available from the publisher's Malden office.

MICROFORM The journal is available on microfilm. For microfilm service, address inquiries to ProQuest Information and Learning, 300 North Zeeb Road, Ann Arbor, MI 48106-1346, USA. Bell and Howell Serials Customer Service Department: 1-800-521-0600 × 2873.

ADVERTISING For information and rates, please visit the journal's website at www.blackwellpublishing.com/journals/MONO email: blackwellads@aidcvt.com, or contact Matt Neckers, Blackwell Advertising Representative, 50 Winter Sport Lane, PO Box 80, Williston, VT 05495. Phone: 800-866-1684 or Fax: 802-864-7749.

POSTMASTER Periodicals class postage paid at Boston, MA, and additional offices. Send address changes to Blackwell Publishing, 350 Main Street, Malden, MA 02148, USA.

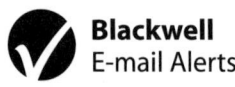

Keep up with new publications from Blackwell Publishing. Join our free e-mail alerting service, and we'll send you journal tables of contents (with links to abstracts) and news of our latest books in your field. Signing up is easy. Simply visit www.blackwellpublishing.com/ealerts. Choose which discipline interests you, and we'll send you a message every other week. OR select exactly which books and journals you'd like to hear about, and when you'd like to receive your messages.

COPYRIGHT All rights reserved. With the exception of fair dealing for the purposes of research or private study, or criticism or review, no part of this publication may be reproduced, stored or transmitted in any form or by any means without the prior permission in writing from the copyright holder. Authorization to photocopy items for internal and personal use is granted by the copyright holder for libraries and other users of the Copyright Clearance Center (CCC), 222 Rosewood Drive, Danvers, MA 01923, USA (www.copyright.com), provided the appropriate fee is paid directly to the CCC. This consent does not extend to other kinds of copying, such as copying for general distribution for advertising or promotional purposes, for creating new collective works or for resale. For all other permissions inquiries, including requests to republish material in another work, please contact the Journals Rights & Permissions Coordinator, Blackwell Publishing, 9600 Garsington Road, Oxford OX4 2DQ, UK. Email: JournalsRights@BlackwellPublishing.com.

© 2003 Society for Research in Child Development

CURRENT

Personal Persistence, Identity Development, and Suicide: A Study of Native and Non-native North American Adolescents—*Michael J. Chandler, Christopher E. Lalonde, Bryan W. Sokol, and Darcy Hallett* (SERIAL NO. 273, 2003)

Personality and Development in Childhood: A Person-Centered Approach—*Daniel Hart, Robert Atkins, and Suzanne Fegley* (SERIAL NO. 272, 2003)

How Children and Adolescents Evaluate Gender and Racial Exclusion—*Melanie Killen, Jennie Lee-Kim, Heidi McGlothlin, and Charles Stangor* (SERIAL NO. 271, 2002)

Child Emotional Security and Interparental Conflict—*Patrick T. Davies, Gordon T. Harold, Marcie C. Goeke-Morey, and E. Mark Cummings* (SERIAL NO. 270, 2002)

The Developmental Course of Gender Differentiation: Conceptualizing, Measuring and Evaluating Constructs and Pathways—*Lynn S. Liben and Rebecca S. Bigler* (SERIAL NO. 269, 2002)

The Development of Mental Processing: Efficiency, Working Memory, and Thinking—*Andreas Demetriou, Constantinos Christou, George Spanoudis, and Maria Platsidou* (SERIAL NO. 268, 2002)

The Intentionality Model and Language Acquisition: Engagement, Effort, and the Essential Tension in Development—*Lois Bloom and Erin Tinker* (SERIAL NO. 267, 2001)

Children with Disabilities: A Longitudinal Study of Child Development and Parent Well-being—*Penny Hauser-Cram, Marji Erickson Warfield, Jack P. Shonkoff, and Marty Wyngaarden Krauss* (SERIAL NO. 266, 2001)

Rhythms of Dialogue in Infancy: Coordinated Timing in Development—*Joseph Jaffe, Beatrice Beebe, Stanley Feldstein, Cynthia L. Crown, and Michael D. Jasnow* (SERIAL NO. 265, 2001)

Early Television Viewing and Adolescent Behavior: The Recontact Study—*Daniel R. Anderson, Aletha C. Huston, Kelly Schmitt, Deborah Linebarger, and John C. Wright* (SERIAL NO. 264, 2001)

Parameters of Remembering and Forgetting in the Transition from Infancy to Early Childhood—*P. J. Bauer, J. A. Wenner, P. L. Dropik, and S. S. Wewerka* (SERIAL NO. 263, 2000)

Breaking the Language Barrier: An Emergentist Coalition Model for the Origins of Word Learning —*George J. Hollich, Kathy Hirsh-Pasek, Roberta Michinick Golinkoff* (SERIAL NO. 262, 2000)

Across the Great Divide: Bridging the Gap Between Understanding of Toddlers' and Other Children's Thinking—*Zhe Chen and Robert Siegler* (SERIAL NO. 261, 2000)

Making the Most of Summer School: A Meta-Analytic and Narrative Review—*Harris Cooper, Kelly Charlton, Jeff C. Valentine, and Laura Muhlenbruck* (SERIAL NO. 260, 2000)

Adolescent Siblings in Stepfamilies: Family Functioning and Adolescent Adjustment—*E. Mavis Hetherington, Sandra H. Henderson, and David Reiss* (SERIAL NO. 259, 1999)

Atypical Attachment in Infancy and Early Childhood Among Children at Developmental Risk—*Joan I. Vondra and Douglas Barnett* (SERIAL NO. 258, 1999)